Returning to Nursing Practice

Returning to Nursing Practice

Confidence and Competence

Ros Wray and Mary Kitson

University of Northampton
Northampton, UK

WILEY Blackwell

Registered Office(s)
John Wiley & Sons, Inc., 111 River Street, Hoboken, NJ 07030, USA
John Wiley & Sons Ltd, The Atrium, Southern Gate, Chichester, West Sussex, PO19 8SQ, UK

Editorial Office
9600 Garsington Road, Oxford, OX4 2DQ, UK

For details of our global editorial offices, customer services, and more information about Wiley products visit us at www.wiley.com.

Wiley also publishes its books in a variety of electronic formats and by print-on-demand. Some content that appears in standard print versions of this book may not be available in other formats.

A catalogue record for this book is available from the Library of Congress

Paperback ISBN: 9781119795872; ePub ISBN: 9781119795889; ePDF ISBN: 9781119795902

Cover image: © Cover image and illustrations by Cecilia Wray
Cover design by Wiley

Set in 10.5/13pt STIXTwoText by Integra Software Services Pvt. Ltd., Pondicherry, India
Printed and bound by CPI Group (UK) Ltd, Croydon, CR0 4YY

C9781119795872_030223

Contents

Preface

Welcome to *Returning to Nursing Practice: Confidence and Competence*. This book is intended as a guide for those contemplating or undertaking a return to their practice role. If you are thinking about going back to your profession after time away, we know that you may also be apprehensive. There may be a sense of lost skills and knowledge, a practice gap that is too wide or a fear that you will not be able to cope with today's working pressures. These are entirely understandable feelings shared by nurses, teachers, social workers and many others. Professional roles such as these are both fulfilling and demanding, carrying at their core ethical responsibilities and a commitment to give to others. There are skills to refresh, knowledge to renew and an identity to reclaim. This is a journey back to confidence and competence. Over twenty years of involvement in supporting returning nurses and health visitors has afforded us insights into what it is like to travel this path. We hope here to both inform and reassure by sharing with you what we have learnt.

Our approach is largely generic across all nursing fields because we wanted to highlight the fact that by far the most significant aspect of returning to professional practice is that it is a shared experience. In some areas our discussions may lean more towards one field than another and, at this point, we must note that we have made only brief mention of midwifery; however, again, as so much of returning to the healthcare professions embraces common ground, we hope returning midwives will find something of value here to take away. Our intention has been to be as inclusive as possible, drawing on and representing examples from across the range of practice specialties.

We have included points of academic reference whilst also aiming to sustain a light flow of reading. We wanted above all to communicate usefully, creating a book which feels friendly and informative. One of the challenges for us has been to find a balance between these two settings, and we hope that this has been achieved. You will find published sources and web links for further reading listed at the end of each chapter. We have endeavoured to be consistent in our terminology, but we are also conscious that returning nurses will have varying orientations to different frames of reference depending on when they were last in practice. As mature nurses we are most comfortable with the term 'patient' to refer to individuals who receive care, and so this is what you will see most often in the text. However, occasionally we have also used 'service user' and 'client'.

There are now a range of routes to choose from when considering a return to nursing. We have outlined these in one of the early chapters. However, our focus is the Return to Practice course because this remains the most popular choice for returning nurses. We believe the reason for this is that students gain invaluably from the support of others embarking on the same journey. Every cohort becomes a small community of fellow travellers who help each other along the way: encouraging, informing, giving each other lifts and often forming solid friendships. They are a courageous, kind and resilient band of individuals and this book pays tribute to their endeavours.

Specifically, we are indebted to the many nurses who have contributed to this book, either directly or indirectly. Their thoughts and feelings have been captured in the Words of Wisdom boxes found throughout the book. Some of these provide a summary of comments from returning students across many cohorts and some reflect the views of individuals. We hope to act as a channel enabling you to hear their voices with the hints, tips and reflections that they have wanted to pass on to you.

The book is organised into eight chapters. We begin with a short opening chapter which addresses the personal decision making involved in a return to nursing. We also consider what nursing identity might mean to us all and set the scene for the start of your journey back to the profession.

Once your decision has been made, Chapter 2 focuses on the practicalities of the next steps. Advice is given about when might be the right time to start a course, with an emphasis on managing self-expectations and maintaining a work-life-study balance. Guidance is provided on course application, course content and placement arrangements. Comparative aspects of community and acute settings are discussed with reference to the four nursing fields and specialist community public health nursing.

Chapter 3 is entitled 'Bridging the gap' referring to the in-between years since a returner last worked as a registered nurse. Returning to practice is first and foremost about regaining confidence. We acknowledge the hopes and fears that individuals often experience when they start the course and highlight the way in which cohorts tend to bond together, offering each other valuable peer support. The chapter focuses on knowing self and the importance of self-assessment and self-efficacy. With growing confidence comes competence, the two going hand in hand throughout the return journey.

Themes crucial to a positive practice experience will be discussed in Chapter 4 including the relationship between the student and supervisor, and the importance of questioning, assertiveness and seeking support. This is a substantial chapter which addresses key areas of contemporary nursing practice such as team working, management and leadership, and clinical judgement. Neither true pre-registration student nurse nor staff nurse, the Return to Practice nurse stands alone; the role is defined as unique and explored with consideration of scope of practice and the importance of understanding your individual practice gap and the value of your professionalism and your prior knowledge and experience.

Whilst detailed coverage of the four nursing fields and Specialist Community Public Health Nursing is beyond the scope of this text, we have explained how field specific nursing competencies and professional standards may be met. The chapter continues by outlining the usual process of assessments along with links to references and resources.

Chapter 5 aims to provide a fresh and rounded view of reflective practice. We hope to re-enthuse those who can only remember reflection as an overused type of assessment, as well as draw the interest of those who are new to the topic. Through the lens of returners' contributions, we consider the significance of stories, self-awareness and the reflective process to ongoing learning and change in nursing practice.

Returning to practice brings both joys and challenges. Studying again after a gap can be frustrating initially because everything feels slow and inaccessible; those first few weeks back in practice can be physically very tiring; and of course, nursing work is emotionally taxing. Suddenly, mind, body and spirit need to work in ways that they may not have done so for some time. In Chapter 6 we suggest a range of tips on how to maintain well-being during your return journey and beyond. Wherever possible, these discussions have been matched to course pinch points so that guidance feels meaningful and relevant.

Many returning nurses feel apprehensive at the prospect of studying again. The gap since they last attended a university can be as much as twenty years, or they may have trained in a school of nursing and therefore not encountered university study before. Chapter 7 acknowledges the diversity of student experience and aims to present some useful advice which will help to strengthen confidence. We hope to convey a sense of how it feels to study again after a break, picking up on key observations and advice that nurse returners have shared with us over the years.

The final chapter marks the completion of the return to practice journey and your arrival back in the professional workforce. Here we celebrate achievement and outline the process of NMC re-registration. We provide some information about preparing for job applications and interviews and share feedback from previous returners about the experience of being back at work.

Our final course day is one of celebration. These are a group of individuals glowing with achievement and sometimes surprised delight at what they have made possible. We have ended the book with their final Words of Wisdom as they share what they have learnt about themselves and prepare to embark on the next stages of their journey. Their stories and experiences have encouraged and enabled us to complete this book and continue our lifelong learning. We hope that it will inspire you with the confidence to undertake your journey back to your professional practice.

Ros Wray and Mary Kitson 2022

Acknowledgements

We are indebted to the many cohorts of returning nurses and health visitors who contributed so generously to the writing of this book. They have been happy to share their written accounts and Words of Wisdom for the benefit of future returners and we could not have achieved this work without their help. We would also like to acknowledge our colleagues for their supportive insights.

Special thanks and acknowledgements go to Ann Walsh, Lindsay Wells, Emma Williams, Gillian Siddall, Valerie Olivant, Michaela Macalister, Lara Lang, Sharon Lock, Tricia James, Chris Jones, Memory Kamhuka, Lisa King, Maria Hames, Susan Hayden, Beverley Hill, Justine Hill, Linda Hoe, Lynne Hoppenbrouwers, Laetitia Gamble, Karen Gibbons, Claire Frisby, Abbie Fordham Barnes, Rebecca Eames, Tracey Dyne, Frances Brookfield and Donna Bray.

We would like to thank Cecilia Wray for her illustrations, and Anne Hunt for her patient guidance.

We are also very grateful for the support and understanding of our close families and friends who have also lived with this project for some considerable time.

CHAPTER 1

Your Time to Return

At any given time, there are thousands of nurses living in the UK who are not actively registered to practise. Many are retired; some will never return, and some are taking a break. Between 2014 and 2021 almost 8,000 nurses did come back to the profession and for each one of these individuals there came a day when they decided to start that journey (Nursing and Midwifery Council (NMC) 2022). In this chapter we will explore the personal decision making involved in a return to nursing. There will be many questions which we hope to be able to go some way to answering. The discussion will highlight practical factors to consider including balancing competing commitments and identifying support networks.

When asked the inevitable question 'Why are you doing this?' many returners talk of a need or pull to come back to nursing. 'It is my turn now', they say. 'I am doing this for me.' Nursing provides many of us with a lasting sense of identity. Our past nursing histories coupled with life experience make a powerful combination (Morton-Cooper 1989). Despite writing over thirty years ago when returning to practice was more of a 'movement' than an established process, Morton-Cooper's words endure, encouraging returners to perceive the value that their nursing skills bring in dealing with everyday challenges and stresses. Years of nursing often leave an individual drawn to the caring of others. Those qualities of listening and responding continue through life whether your professional registration is lapsed or active. Your nursing knowledge and skills may be out of date, but your impulse to care is likely to be as strong as ever. In addition, your sense of professionalism and your ability to assess and plan will also be alive and well. You will know that once a nurse always a nurse. All that remains is for you to find the confidence and competence to become again a safe and contemporary practitioner.

YOUR NURSING IDENTITY

Your reasons for wanting to return may echo those first questions we can all remember being asked at interview about our choice of nursing as a career. Why do you want to be a nurse? What qualities do you possess that will help you to be a nurse? For many, responses tend to be based on caring principles and the desire to make a difference. The concept of care is one of the most important aspects of nursing. A positive correlation has been identified between intrinsic factors such as caring, helping and taking responsibility for others and the decision to become a nurse (Ben Natan and Becker 2010). Clearly differentiated from the 'curing' focus of the medical profession, nursing has traditionally been associated with 'caring' with nurses viewing care as a major part of who they are (Traynor and Evans 2014).

Words of Wisdom

Returning to professional practice is personally and professionally challenging. Our identities as nurses are shaped by our initial experiences of nurse education and our subsequent careers are equally shaped by the culture and practices we encounter. Returning to the register involves a leap of faith; will what we know and remember matter? Will we adapt and succeed as evidence-based practitioners? My own experience of Return to Practice was both humbling and liberating. My practice placement valued my experience, and my university tutor challenged me to think differently. Returning to the register allowed me to review my professional identity and rejoin the nursing family. I hope those who take this route feel as inspired and reinvigorated as I did.

A sense of professional identity starts to develop during our nurse education when we discover what caring means. As we progress and our knowledge grows, our core nursing values integrate with skills of communication and clinical reasoning. We think and feel and behave as a nurse. Although it may wax and wane through our lives, this sense of being never leaves us. Professional identity develops and evolves at different stages throughout working life (Tamm 2010; Bridges 2018). It is shaped and monitored by a professional code and defined by individual attitudes, beliefs and values. Bridges (2018) suggests that our professional identity relates predominantly to integrity, compassion and person-centeredness. These remain the core values of the nursing profession despite the changes in training and education as we journey into the 21st century. What patients cherish and remember most is kindness, empathy and compassion (NHS England/ Nursing Directorate 2013). As you would expect, these qualities continue to be championed in the NMC Code and nursing standards (NMC 2018a, 2018b). As a team we have personal experience of the trepidation commonly felt on returning to the clinical environment after a gap in practice. However, whilst the variations in technology, systems and processes will always present initial challenges, most significant is the fact that patients' needs remain unchanged.

> ## Words of Wisdom from a Returning Nurse on Starting a New Job
>
> Having been in my role for four months I wake up every morning and look forward to going to work in the knowledge that I am making a difference to the lives of the patients in my care.

THE STARTING POINT

Returners will often talk about the point in time when they started to contemplate coming back to practice. For some, nursing a loved one has reawakened a sense of needing to care more widely again; for others, the frustrations of not feeling fulfilled by a current occupation may have sparked a sudden insight. Perhaps a chance conversation with a former nursing colleague has triggered memories. Some have always planned their return, perhaps to coincide with when their children commence school or when a family commitment is lifted; and some returning nurses have been surprised by the urge to respond to a perceived need, even if that means coming out of retirement.

> ## Words of Wisdom
>
> In December 2010 I took premature retirement from my nursing career due to organisational reconfiguration. At the time this was quite a life-changing move as it was something unexpected and not how I had planned my career would progress. For more than thirty years I had been passionate about people, patients and their care but at this time I remember the juxtaposition of feeling guilty for 'letting people down' and wounded as a casualty of NHS change.
>
> My new situation allowed me the opportunity to realise a long-held ambition to own a restaurant and this was my focus for seven years. However, during this time I also needed to care for a poorly relative and this was the point at which I started to inwardly question my decision to leave nursing. Providing twenty-four-hour care helped to confirm my views that nursing was for me always a natural vocation. The positive impact that nurses can have on someone else's life is an inspiring role to deliver.
>
> In February 2019 I returned to a caring role and then reflecting upon professional and social responsibility I also joined the army of people in the fight against COVID-19. Becoming a vaccinator was predicated upon the achievement of nationally prescribed competencies and at the time I remember questioning whether I still had the skill, knowledge and mental agility to succeed. Thankfully I overcame my apprehension and that, together with support from my colleagues, gave me the confidence to consider returning to practice.

> On one occasion at the vaccination centre, I was asked about my previous work history and replied that I had been a nurse. My colleague responded by saying 'once a nurse, always a nurse'. Whilst this may not be true for everyone, it certainly has proved to be the case for me, and I have now successfully regained my registration.

Global shortages in the healthcare workforce had prompted the World Health Organisation (WHO 2020) to designate 2020 as the year of the nurse and midwife. This acknowledgement and celebration of these important roles was intended to raise the profile of the profession and advocate for additional investment. Unfortunately, the initiative was overshadowed by the COVID-19 pandemic which continues to challenge all aspects of society and healthcare provision across the world (Moynihan et al. 2020).

Despite the destabilising effects of so much of our day-to-day life including family relationships, travel, education, working practices and supply chains, nurses rose to meet the needs of those most vulnerable, adapting practice and protocols to provide care throughout. New ways of working and organising care were swiftly put into place. Vindrola-Padros et al. (2020) highlight that supportive work environments are crucial for motivating staff during times of challenge; without the usual bureaucratic red tape, practice can be modified and adapted very quickly. The NMC temporary registrar is a good example of this response. Thousands of nurses who had left the register through retirement or change in career were urged to return to the workforce to utilise their experience and skills and be part of the NHS COVID-19 workforce. The NMC temporary register opened in March 2020 and was still recording over 13,000 active nurses in August 2021 (NMC 2021a). This upsurge in returning nurses to the workforce during the pandemic is testament to lifelong passion and dedication to the profession.

The COVID-19 pandemic has also put a spotlight on nursing as a career. Applications to study nursing have risen by a third not just from school leavers but also from older adults seeking a change in career direction (UCAS 2022). This is positive news in the face of an overall decline in UK nursing numbers: 11.3% of registered nurses (around 27,000) left the profession in 2021 (NMC 2022). Demographic figures are also a cause for concern as within the next few years it is anticipated that an increasing number of registered nurses will be eligible to retire. Current workforce analysis predicts that the current shortfall of 50,000 nurses could rise to nearly 64,000 by 2024 (The Health Foundation 2022).

Subsequently, more investment is proposed in the NHS workforce with training of health professionals across all sectors. Attention has also been paid to the working conditions of NHS staff with the launch of the People Plan in 2020/2021, set up to encourage a more inclusive supportive work environment. We will return to this subject in our chapter on well-being.

WHY DID YOU LEAVE?

> ### Words of Wisdom
>
> I feel I need to say how I came to leave nursing originally. My main reason was my young family at the time, with it often being difficult to manage being there for them as I had no alternative childcare available. This has improved vastly since but, although not going back to nursing was one of the hardest decisions, it felt the best option for us as a family. I had considered returning to nursing a few years before and even made enquiries with the course leaders. However, I continued to put off taking it further as my family always seemed to need me. I have realised now that they are always going to need me, but as they have become teens and young adults, they also need that increased independence. The year I finally made the decision to return was the pandemic of COVID-19. I felt frustrated that I was not in the nursing workforce with having skills and knowledge that could have helped my colleagues and patients at their crisis point. I suppose COVID-19 was a catalyst in my decision to return.

It may help to think back to when you last nursed. Were you working in the acute sector, or were you community-based? If you were a single person with few commitments, a demanding and fast-paced job may have felt exciting and rewarding; however, if you now have a family and an elderly parent to support, you may feel that a slower or less acute environment would suit you better. Many nurses leave the profession for family reasons, whilst others may move into a managerial role or a different career entirely. Statistics show that whilst nursing registers as one of the most rewarding jobs, it also carries a heavy emotional burden. It may be that a past nursing role prompts memories of strain and fatigue. In 2014 a literature review carried out by Health Education England (HEE) acknowledged that the most common cause of nurses leaving the National Health Service was work-related stress (HEE 2014). It is important to reflect on your time as a nurse and to ask yourself what you valued most, and what was difficult to cope with? These are vital considerations which will help guide your direction of travel as you think about your return to the profession. Sustaining and balancing your well-being as a nurse is fundamental to a successful return to the profession and we will be looking at this in detail in Chapter 6.

IS IT THE RIGHT TIME TO RETURN?

Judging when to return requires careful thinking and planning. Many nurses leave the profession to have children. The start of full-time education for children can mark a significant transition for all family members, and it can provide parents with the opportunity to return to careers. However, with good childcare in place, it may be possible to consider returning when a child starts nursery. It is important to tune into what feels right for all concerned; this may mean reviewing how existing arrangements could be expanded or modified to accommodate your plans. We would advise that you talk to your family about what might be possible and look further afield to see who else may be happy to help.

It is possible to get the timing wrong. We remember one applicant who desperately wanted to come back to nursing, but who arrived for an informal chat with three young children in tow, all under the age of five. She did have some child-care in place and willing parents to hand, but as we talked through the course and placement requirements, she began to see a reality of rushed journeys to and from practice, school and childminders and evenings torn between studying and bedtimes. It was too early. She left disappointed. However, she did succeed in returning to nursing a few years later when able to balance her personal commitments more comfortably. The next section examines issues related to family and young children in more detail.

You will need to allocate nine months to a year when planning your return journey. Traditional Return to Practice courses can range in length from four to six months, and you will need to factor in additional time for application and re-registration processes. This does not mean that everything else in your life is on hold; but it

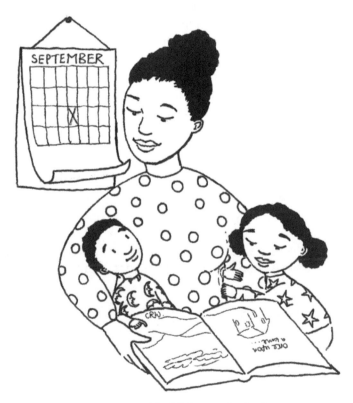

ILLUSTRATION NO. 1.1 Young mum with children and calendar.

does mean, that returning to practice will dominate. Most courses are part time (although they may not feel like it!), so a short holiday can usually be accommodated alongside. Any protracted time away, though, is best scheduled for the future. Similarly, if you have a part-time job with fixed days or hours, this may well be difficult to fit with days in placement where matching your Practice Supervisor's shifts must take precedence for review and assessment of your practice to be feasible. Flexible part-time work and an understanding employer can be a supportive element in your return to nursing, especially if the work is healthcare related but it does require negotiation and transparency to avoid any potential conflict of interest from the existing employer.

Some courses are run several times each year, so it is well worth inquiring about different intakes if you do have an important commitment to work around. Many students opt to avoid the school holidays, preferring to commence a course in the autumn or spring. Planning in this way will ensure a smoother and less stressful experience.

WHAT HAVE YOU BEEN DOING SINCE YOU STOPPED NURSING?

Return to Practice students come with a wide variability in background. Some may possess little or no post-registration experience whilst others will have occupied senior clinical or management roles. You may have left nursing to pursue an alternative career or job. This is not uncommon. We have spoken to and supported returners who have started up businesses, become teachers or researchers, or taken up charity work. Their reasons for wanting to nurse again are of course multi-faceted, but many share a sense of incomplete fulfilment and a pull to contribute again within a purely caring role. Here is one returner's story:

Words of Wisdom

I initially qualified as a nurse in the late 1980s and spent twenty-seven years wearing my uniform with pride. I qualified as an independent nurse prescriber, specialised as an urgent care practitioner and became a trainer and assessor for post-graduate nurses undertaking level 6 university training. In 2014, I had the opportunity to train as a Special Constable, volunteering in my community as a police officer. I found this extremely rewarding and made the decision in 2017 to change careers. I left the NHS and joined the police as a regular full-time police officer. I was happy in my role, serving as a front-line officer.

In 2019 the world changed with the arrival of COVID-19.... Many of my friends were still working as nurses and under enormous pressure. In late 2020 the 'call to arms' was made by the government to support the vaccine programme and I joined the NMC temporary nursing register. This allowed me to support the NHS, becoming a COVID-19 vaccinator and doing my bit to help my community. I requested a three-year career break from my role as a police officer to support the COVID-19 vaccination programme. This was granted with full support. I then made the decision that I wanted to reinstate my NMC registration.

I was fortunate to join the Return to Practice nursing course with Northampton University. The course was rewarding, and I particularly enjoyed the opportunity to reflect on my past and recent nursing practice. I successfully completed my course last year. I am now happy to be back in the NHS, working within the learning and development team as a clinical educator. I currently have no plans to return to the police. I would highly recommend the Return to Practice programme and hope my story has inspired you to re-join the nursing profession.

Healthcare assistant work can provide a useful platform from which to launch a return to nursing. Whether you are hospital or community-based, this role will bring you up to date with healthcare teams and settings and, most importantly, put you back in touch with patient care. It is crucial, though, to balance any work commitments with the demands of the course so that student hours and employed hours are co-ordinated, separate and well-paced.

Learning and teaching assistant work in schools is also favoured by nurses with lapsed registration. This role has relevance to parenting, and caring in a wider context, and may enable some to use their nursing experience as first aiders or within special needs. It provides a good precursor to returning to practice. Again, though, it is vital to negotiate a flexible working pattern whilst undertaking your clinical placement. For some returnees this may not be possible, and they may decide to resign their post before commencing the course.

Some individuals have remained in the healthcare sector but progressed their careers into management posts. They may have reached a point of needing to renew a lost connection with patients in clinical settings. If this is you, be prepared for those around you in your practice placement to soon perceive this wealth of experience, even if it is not obvious to you! You may feel that others expect you to perform at a higher level than feels comfortable or, more likely, you may expect this of yourself. Every returner will have challenges to manage; for those who have been used to a senior role in the past, the task may be to reset expectations and present yourself as a student who needs to learn and feel supported. Once you have found your feet and your own comfort level, you will be able to move forward with growing confidence. When you return to the nursing workforce you will initially find yourself in a more junior role again. Some welcome this and have no urge to return to management; others will find that their knowledge and skills takes them inevitably in that direction.

Occasionally returners join the course with no post-registration experience prior to their break. Often this is a result of individual personal circumstances. Following qualification and registration, one recent student was unable to take up a post because he was needed to care full-time for an elderly relative who had become suddenly unwell. However, he was able to secure an employment route for his return to nursing in an area where he was already working as a Healthcare Assistant. The benefits of working and learning in a team of known colleagues brought a sense of belonging and helped him to build the confidence required for his future role as a registered nurse.

THE TEST OF COMPETENCE: AN ALTERNATIVE ROUTE TO RE-REGISTRATION

You may feel overwhelmed with the thought of undertaking a course of study and spending a protracted time in a placement under supervision. It may be that no university in your area runs the course, or the logistics and timeframes may be impossible. Perhaps your registration has recently lapsed without you intending it to do so. In recent years, the NMC have tightened up their time allowances for re-registration, and this has inevitably caused some issues with nurses who for one reason or another – be it ill health, moving to a new house or caring for another – have been unable to meet the strict criteria for renewing registration and meeting revalidation requirements. Besides the traditional course route, it has been determined in recent years and highlighted in the new RTP standards that another route to re-entry to the register is needed to provide greater flexibility and acknowledge the value of nurses returning to the profession (NMC 2019; Scammell 2019). The Test of Competence (ToC) offers an outcomes-based route which is consistent and standardised and was initially introduced by the NMC in 2014 for internationally qualified nurses and midwives. In 2018 it became an option for UK registered nurses as a route to return to practice.

The ToC option has been channelled as a new pathway which assesses clinical skill and competence in real-world scenarios. It is a relatively new option for nurses returning to the register; it may suit some more than others. Nurses with lapsed registration, who contributed their service via a temporary register during the COVID-19 pandemic, may now find that the ToC provides a fast track to return to the profession. It can offer a speedier process and may appeal especially to those whose registration has recently lapsed and who still feel broadly confident in their knowledge base and in the prospect of performing skills under scrutiny.

There are two components to the test, and it is available across the four fields of nursing and midwifery.

- Part 1 is a computer-based test (CBT) consisting of two parts – one clinical and one numeracy. The numeracy test consists of fifteen questions based on medication dosages and infusion/fluid balance calculations. The clinical section is a multiple-choice quiz which combines a clinical focus with overlapping generic questions for different fields of nursing. Part 1 is available in most countries throughout the world and can be accessed via a Pearson VUE test centre. It is possible to take the test in any order although nurses from overseas tend to take Part 1 first in their home country and then proceed to Part 2 once authorised by the NMC.
- Part 2 is the Objective Structured Clinical Examination (OSCE). This is designed to test candidates' ability to assess, plan, implement and evaluate care based on

everyday practice scenarios. The test is only accessible in designated test centres in the UK. Currently, there are four test centres in the UK: these are located at the University of Northampton, Oxford Brookes University, Ulster University and Northumbria University.

It is possible to sit the CBT or the OSCE in any order but both components must be successfully completed within two years. The application process is through the NMC and there are links and resources freely available via the NMC website or alternative providers to support and prepare for the tests. Preparation materials include mock OSCEs, webinars and reading materials, information booklets, marking criteria and examples of the relevant documentation used such as observation charts.

The scenarios are structured so that you can apply your knowledge and skills to demonstrate person-centred care and best practice. The OSCE is made up of ten stations some of which are scenario-based and related to the nursing process framework: assessment, planning, implementation and evaluation. There are also two sets of three stations which test linked skills and two written stations assessing professional values and critical appraisal of evidence and decision making. Communication is fundamental to nursing practice and is assessed throughout the scenarios.

The ToC is designed to ensure you are a safe competent practitioner at the point of registration. The knowledge and skills assessed are aligned to the Future Nurse Standards (NMC 2018b) which are generic and apply across all fields of nursing: adult nursing, mental health, child and learning disabilities. This reflects the complexity of today's nursing with many patients having co-morbidities that require highly skilled input from specialists from a range of disciplines.

This route can be pursued independently or with support from employers. Some Trusts offer employment routes for returning to the register; this may be an area worth exploring locally. There can be contractual requirements with this offer with some organisations proposing employment as a Healthcare Assistant for a set number of working hours in conjunction with supporting you through the ToC. This can be beneficial if you have not quite made up your mind about re-entering the register; the opportunity to work in a supported and supervised healthcare setting may give you the confidence you need to make this decision.

The employment-led approach can also work alongside the traditional Return to Practice course and for some students the chance to earn whilst undertaking the course is very beneficial. However, if this route is of interest and available, do be mindful of the contractual requirements as you may find combining working hours with the additional responsibilities of completing the programme demanding.

Both the ToC and RTP course options are available to returners to date, and it is up to the individual to choose which route suits their needs best. Both are professionally regulated by the NMC with information about where and how to apply accessible on the NMC website (NMC 2021b). The NMC and Health Education England websites also provide case studies from previous returning students so do take time to browse and get a sense of what both routes entail. It is important to weigh up the pros and cons before deciding. Currently it is not possible to update a Specialist Community and Public Health Nursing (SCPHN) registration via this route; however, specialist practice qualifications including SCPHN are under review by the NMC and so this may become an alternative option going forward.

FINANCIAL ISSUES

Any change in direction in life or career can be challenging. Family finance was identified by the NMC as one of the main barriers to re-joining the register with 58% of returners citing it as a concern (NMC 2019). It is a difficult decision to make particularly with rising household costs and, of course, a matter for individuals to work out income and expenditure to see where and if adjustments can be made. The usual practical tips apply including setting a limit on spending, checking tax codes and benefit eligibility – all things which may help draw additional income in the short term.

Return to practice courses have been government funded as a part of a wider workforce recruitment strategy. This means that your course fees will be funded by HEE, the organisation responsible for the education and development of the healthcare workforce (Health Education England 2014). You will also be provided with a payment to help cover some of your travel costs and expenses whilst undertaking the course. Details of this funding can be found on the HEE website along with a variety of resources which provide a very good starting point if you are returning to the profession.

Since 2014 HEE has been instrumental in supporting almost 8,000 nurses back into the workforce (HEE 2021). The vision of HEE is to supply the NHS with a skilled and competent NHS workforce to meet demand to ensure safe patient outcomes. Their wider strategy aims to develop systems which enable the range of allied health professionals to return to practice and this, of course, is crucial to maintain safe staffing levels. Circumstances can change with governments fluctuating from funding to non-funding according to the times. The prospect of a funded course is an important incentive for those individuals coming back to the workforce following time out with family; for others already in employment, making the transition back to a period of education could result in a temporary income shortfall.

THINKING AHEAD

Whatever your background, it can be helpful at this early stage to have some thoughts as to your future career direction. A long-term goal – such as moving from nursing to health visiting – will require some stepping-stones. In this instance, your first thoughts may be on updating your acute nursing skills through a ward-based placement which reflects your previous experience. Following re-registration, you may then decide to spend twelve months working in inpatient general medicine to build further confidence and consolidate your nursing skills before perhaps taking a community nursing role with a health visiting team. It would then be an additional step to undertake your health visiting training.

You may not yet know what you want to do once back on the register. Some returners are happy to look around gauging their thoughts and feelings with 'a toe in the water' before deciding on their next move. For many, the notion of a big career plan may not chime with current thinking or circumstances; self-fulfilment may be about returning to the heart of the nursing role, caring again for patients and enjoying the camaraderie of a nursing team. Job opportunities will arise whilst you are on the course, and we would encourage you to pursue those of interest; remember that your time in practice placements will also enable informal conversations about potential vacancies. Most employers are keen to recruit returners who they know have much to offer and whose progress back to professional competence they have been able to follow. Interviews and appointments often happen during the course with provision for interim roles to cover the period between successful course completion and NMC re-registration. There is, therefore, no wrong time to apply for posts: the message is that once enrolled on your course, the job market is open.

This could be something that you have toyed with for a long time either as a closely guarded secret or as a threat to errant teenagers! It may be that your circumstances have changed, and this is a decision that has come about sooner than you anticipated. Whatever your reason, a return to nursing is a major decision but also a frequently travelled path. Hopefully, we will be able to provide some insight and practical advice as you make your journey. We can also reassure you will not be alone – others will be travelling with you!

REFERENCES

Ben Natan, M. and Becker, F. (2010). Israelis' perceived motivation for choosing a nursing career. *Nurse Education Today* 30 (4): 308–313.

Bridges, S.J. (2018). Professional identity development: learning and journeying together. *Research in Social and Administrative Pharmacy* 14 (3): 290–294.

Health Education England (2014). *Literature review on nurses leaving the NHS*. Health Education England. website https://www.hee.nhs.uk.

The Health Foundation (2022). *REAL centre Projections*. https://www.health.org.uk/publications/nhs-workforce-projections-2022.

HEE (2021). https://www.hee.nhs.uk/news-blogs-events/news/nurses-midwives-offered-increased-incentive-return-practice.

Morton-Cooper, A. (1989). *Returning to Nursing. A Guide for Nurses and Health Visitors*. London: Macmillan Education Ltd.

Moynihan, R., Johannsson, M., Maybee, A. et al. (2020). Covid-19: an opportunity to reduce unnecessary healthcare. *British Medical Journal* 370: m2752. https://www.bmj.com/content/bmj/370/bmj.m2752.full.pdf (accessed 3rd May 2022).

NHS England /Nursing Directorate (2013). *Compassion in Practice: One Year On*. NHS England.

NMC (2018b). *Future Nurse: Standards of Proficiency for Registered Nurses*. NMC.

NMC (2019). *Part 3: Standards for Return to Practice Programmes*. NMC

NMC (2021a). https://www.nmc.org.uk/news/news-and-updates/nmc-register-data-september-2021.

NMC (2021b). Test of Competence 2021 for nurses and midwives. https://www.nmc.org.uk/registration/joining-the-register/toc/toc-2021.

NMC (2022). *The NMC register: annual registration data report*. nmc.org.uk.

Nursing and Midwifery Council (NMC) (2018a). *The Code. Professional Standards of Practice and Behaviour for Nurses, Midwives and Nursing Associates*. NMC.

Scammell, J. (2019). Back to nursing: new standards for return to practice programmes. *British Journal of Nursing* 28 (11).

Tamm, T. (2010). *Professional Identity and Self-concept of Estonian Social Workers*. Tampere University Press.

Traynor, M. and Evans, A. (2014). Slavery and jouissance: analysing complaints of suffering in UK and Australian nurses' talk about their work. *Nursing Philosophy* 15 (3): 192–200.

UCAS (2022). https://www.ucas.com/corporate/news-and-key-documents/news/pandemic-inspires-future-nurses-welcome-increase-school-and-college-leavers-looking-enter-profession.

Vindrola-Padros, C., Chisnall, G., Cooper, S. et al. (2020). Carrying out rapid qualitative research during a pandemic: emerging lessons from COVID-19. *Qualitative Health Research* 30 (14): 2192–2204.

World Health Organization (2020). Year of the nurse and the midwife 2020.

CHAPTER 2

Preparation

Once you have made the decision to return to nursing, planning is crucial. The first step is to gauge your current set of circumstances. You will need to weigh external and internal factors so that you have a clear picture of where to most channel your energies. An initial quick self-inquiry may help you to shape your preparations. Here are some questions that may be helpful:

- What roles do I now have in life?
- Does this differ to when I last nursed?
- What and who will help me?
- What type of nursing am I most familiar with?
- Where do I want to be in a year's time?
- What are my strengths?
- What could be a potential source of difficulty?

CURRENT ROLES AND COMMITMENTS

A role can be defined as 'a position or purpose that someone has in a situation, organisation, society or relationship' (Cambridge English Dictionary 2022). Roles in life span the breadth of our human experience, appearing in cultural, social and work contexts. They can evolve, develop, intertwine and disappear. Some may be lifelong such as our gender or being a sibling; some are more temporary and situation-specific such as acting as an eyewitness or an interviewer. Once we accept or acquire a role,

Returning to Nursing Practice: Confidence and Competence, First Edition. Ros Wray and Mary Kitson.
© 2023 John Wiley & Sons Ltd. Published 2023 by John Wiley & Sons Ltd.

we also take on the responsibilities that come with it. So, for example, if you have agreed to work in a charity shop for four hours every week, you have an obligation to comply with the requirements of that position. It could be argued that mature working adults tend to have the most roles and therefore perform the most juggling! The key, of course, is to be aware of how many roles you have so that you can avoid the strain that can arise when they become overloaded or conflicted (Creary and Gordon 2016).

A useful exercise is to write down your current roles and obligations. It may look something like this:

- Parent
- Spouse/partner
- Sibling
- Daughter/son to elderly parent
- Home maker
- Part-time charity worker
- Neighbour
- Friend
- Dog owner
- Jogger

When you commence your return to practice journey, you will be adding 'student' to your list. It is essential, therefore, to weigh and review your commitments so that you can maintain a workable balance. For example, you may have housework to do, a two-day per week part-time job with one fixed day on Fridays, two school age children, a large dog and a disabled brother living locally who you visit twice weekly. Add returning to practice and that comes to six roles! You could find yourself quite pressurised if you try to fulfil all these commitments in the usual way. However, a few tweaks and some planning could make all the difference. You decide to prioritise study time over some house-working chores such as ironing and arrange for your children to walk the dog on Fridays, visiting your brother en route. Streamlining roles can also initiate permanent changes, unclogging over-laborious everyday routines which may have become habitual for you, but which could present new and exciting responsibilities for others. One student explained to us that when she stopped cooking most meals from scratch, preferring convenience food which would free up more study evenings, her teenage son took over the job perfecting a weekly curry which has now become his specialty!

Another way of acknowledging your current situation is to compare it with when you last worked as a registered nurse. You will have been younger and perhaps had more free time. It is important to think this through because, whilst it is unlikely to alter your motivation to return, it may help you to plan what kind of nursing post would best fit your life now. Night shifts in an acute setting may not now be feasible; however, four days a week in day surgery or a community nursing team may be an attractive prospect.

THE RETURN TO PRACTICE COURSE

> **Course provider perspective**
>
> Universities have many years of experience in delivering Return to Practice courses. Our commitment to these learners is very clear. We understand the reasons why nurses may both leave and wish to return to the professional register. Providing a route to return respects the value and privilege we attach to supporting this valuable group of people. Understanding the needs of returning nurses requires a supportive and individualised educational approach. The benefit to employers and service users of a nurse with lived experience and new knowledge re-joining the profession is reason enough to offer these unique programmes of study.

Since the 1990s the traditional route of return to the profession has been via a Return to Practice course, and most nurse returners still choose this option. Courses offer structure, peer support and a process of time enabling adjustment and re-orientation; they also have low attrition rates with most students achieving successful completion and with good prospects of progressing on to jobs. They do require commitment and may not be the best option for nurses who have only recently lapsed on the register and therefore may feel able to fast track re-entry via the Test of Competence (HEE 2014).

University courses can cater for returners from all four nursing fields, and from specialist community public health nursing and midwifery. The mix nearly always reflects the workforce with adult returners constituting the majority nursing field in any group. However, provision is made for each student to follow their own personalised journey with specialist input from senior lecturers from mental health and learning disabilities nursing, children's nursing and health visiting or school nursing. Cohorts tend to be relatively small and therefore provide opportunities for friendships to form with individuals from a range of backgrounds. There is much to share along the way. The value of peer support cannot be over-estimated and is probably the single most important aspect of returning to practice. Here is how one returning health visitor recalls her first few days on the course:

> **Words of Wisdom**
>
> Initial feelings included fear of not being accepted by my peer group. However, I needn't have worried. The other students on the course were a group of nurses from various nursing backgrounds with a wealth of knowledge and skills who were all emotionally supportive of each other whenever we were in university together. We all joined a social media group to extend the support to each other online – after all we all had a common goal.

APPLICATION

Most higher education courses require online applications and Return to Practice is no exception. If this prospect feels like your first obstacle, do enlist some help. Most of us know someone with good IT skills. To match the pace of computer technology, these valuable people are constant learners and therefore often happy to assist others. Children also are a good source of support because many have been introduced to computers at an early age and are not fearful of making mistakes. With all that said, some online course processes can be tricky, requiring you to complete complex forms and upload a variety of documents. Rather than grappling alone with an unfamiliar problem, we would advise that you contact University Admissions teams or course lecturers either by telephone or email. Not only will they be able to guide you through, but it may also reveal a glitch in the system that can then be addressed for the benefit of other applicants.

Words of Wisdom

I did find gathering all the information required to apply to the course a challenge. I required help with some of the technology, so my daughters assisted as this was another area I had hardly used during my years away from work.

ENTRY REQUIREMENTS

Entry requirements for UK Return to Practice courses hinge on evidence of previous nursing registration with the NMC (NMC 2019). This comes in the form of your NMC Personal Identification Number (PIN). This number remains the same as the original but it will appear 'ghosted out' on NMC records to indicate a lapsed registration. As part of your course application, you will be asked to provide your NMC PIN usually via a current NMC Statement of Entry. This document can be accessed via the NMC website and gives details of your registration status much in the way a bank statement provides information of current funds. It is important that the details are correct. Any relationship status changes must be communicated; the NMC may delay re-activation of your registration if their records do not match up. As is now the case with many organisations, the NMC conducts much of its business electronically so you may be able to update your records online.

Some applicants may have Fitness to Practice issues, recorded as sanctions by the NMC. The need to assure public safety lies at the heart of all NMC regulatory procedures. A nurse's practice can be called into question for different reasons including not undertaking care competently or suspicion of dishonesty or fraud. The NMC investigate Fitness to Practice cases and have the power to impose sanctions, the most serious of which is a striking off order resulting in the individual concerned not being allowed to continue to practise as a nurse. After a period of usually five years, this order may be reviewed by the NMC who can then grant a restoration order pending successful completion of a Return to Practice programme.

If you have this kind of background, you will naturally feel anxious about sharing it with course lecturers and admission teams. However, it is imperative that you demonstrate honesty and openness by fully disclosing what has occurred. Your course team will follow a formal process requesting documentary evidence of any NMC hearings and recommendations. It is vital that you are forthcoming and compliant because your response will form part of the ultimate decision as to whether you can proceed with your course application. Very often, a full disclosure along with clear signs that you have reflected on and learnt from the events will be sufficient to convince course teams that you deserve a course place. They will be looking for genuine evidence of the professional values and integrity that underpin high standards of nursing practice as set out in the Code (NMC 2018).

Disclosure and Barring Service (DBS)

In addition to proof of NMC PIN, Return to Practice applicants will be asked to provide an enhanced Disclosure and Barring Service check (DBS) to demonstrate their good character. Nursing courses require an enhanced police check which usually covers the preceding five years. Whilst this application process has been streamlined, it can still take time, so it is important to get things underway as soon as possible. This can be problematic for individuals who have lived abroad as foreign checks can take a long time to arrive and, in some cases, may even result in an applicant having to defer to a later course intake.

If you are worried about something that is recorded on your DBS certificate it is again crucial that you disclose this to the course team. Universities will follow due process in compliance with their formal policies and procedures maintaining confidentiality and ensuring that you are afforded the opportunity to provide information about the matter. Again, transparency, honesty and a sense of remorse will weigh favourably. A gap in years between the recorded crime and the present day will also help to demonstrate positive learning and a commitment to enduring behaviour changes. The applicant is responsible for disclosing any issues to the potential placement provider who will ultimately make the final decision. What must also be made clear is that even if you go on to complete the course successfully, the NMC still reserve the right to disallow your application to re-enter the nursing register on the grounds of your positive criminal record. In practice, we have only experienced this happen on one or two occasions; however, delays are common as the NMC will take steps to follow their own inquiries until they are satisfied that re-registration poses no undue risk to public safety.

Occupational Health Checks

Fitness to practice is also about good physical and mental health. You will need to complete an Occupational Health check as part of your return to practice application. This process is usually accessed initially online and then followed up with a face-to-face appointment at a designated Occupational Health department. The key purpose of course is to ensure that you are cleared as fit and healthy before re-entering clinical settings, and this starts with checking your immunity status. Often, returning practitioners will require boosters before they can start their practice placements. Some may have long-term conditions such as arthritis, asthma or mental health issues, and so the health check also assesses how well these are managed, and whether 'reasonable adjustments' will need to be put in place to support the individual. When such measures are needed, course teams will take time to explore suitable strategies with the student concerned. One response might be to create a plan setting out how supportive steps can be adopted in placement. Plans are reviewed regularly to ensure that they are effective and reasonable.

LEARNING DIFFERENCES

In a similar way, it is also important to communicate any learning differences that you feel may have an impact on your studies. It is known that many adults have learnt to work around undiagnosed or known dyslexia, creating their own strategies to mitigate the difficulties of negotiating a world so heavily reliant on the written word. Indeed, there are a range of simple measures such as highlighting text, using visual materials and listening to the spoken word which can be helpful to all students. We all have individual preferences when it comes to studying, and in a later chapter we will explore this area in more detail. If you know that you are dyslexic or have an alternative confirmed learning difference or neurodivergence, please do let course teams know so that they can help you to access the comprehensive resources and support available in universities. It may be just a question of reminding yourself of what works for you. If you have always wondered why it takes you longer than others to complete a reading task, or why you prefer to listen to audio feedback rather than scan emails, it may be worth going for screening and assessment. The process can take time, however, so this is something to set in motion early. The reality may be that learning support may not come in time for your return to practice course, but it will be there to assist you with future studies. A link for the British Dyslexia Association can be found at the end of this chapter.

PROFESSIONALISM

Before you start your Return to Practice journey, we would advise you to think carefully about your social media. During your 'gap' years digital platforms may have become more integrated into your daily life, giving rise to increasing complexity when it comes to managing your online activity. Your attentiveness in this area may have faded whilst out of nursing practice. Now is the time to set yourself some ground rules regarding responsible posting. An email address such as twinklewhitefairydust@yahoo.com may sound amusing but does not lend itself to a professional image. Remember that any information, comments or photos that appear on popular platforms including Twitter, Facebook and Instagram are permanent. Restricting parameters may give a sense of false security as to who can view this information but ultimately it is out there in the public domain. It is important to ensure that you reflect professional values and behaviours in both the virtual domain and the real world. The NMC has specific guidance on using social media responsibly which may be worth reviewing (NMC 2016).

ADMISSION DAYS AND INTERVIEWS

The application process may require you to provide written information in the form of a personal statement. Course teams will be interested to read about your past nursing experience and understand your motivation to return to the profession. Literacy skills and English language ability are assessed, so do take time and care when completing written statements. Once you have completed the application process, it is likely that you will be called for interview. Again, you may be asked to submit written responses to pre-interview questions.

The interview day will vary considerably in format depending on individual university processes. It may be online or face-to-face; you could find yourself mixing and socialising with other applicants or negotiating access to a virtual shared space. If the day is online and you are unfamiliar with the use of software platforms, try not to let this put you off. Most work via a step-by-step process and there is always help on hand if you experience problems. On occasions connectivity can be an issue for everyone including the interviewers, so do persevere and remember that a quick email to the course team will alert them to any difficulties.

There will be an opportunity to speak privately at some point during the day and the actual interview is likely to be a one-to-one experience with course teams at pains to maintain confidentiality. Remember that most prospective returners are successful in gaining course places, so try not to be too nervous. It is just as important for you to decide whether this is the right course for you as it is for your interviewers to make a judgement about your suitability so do make sure that you have all your questions answered.

Words of Wisdom

When I was invited for an online interview, I was so pleased I had made it this far, although a few hours before my interview my youngest daughter had a positive COVID-19 test result. I certainly will have my interview day etched on my memory! The interviewers made me feel at my ease and were very encouraging with their response to my answers. One hurdle to face when returning was having a suitable placement, as they ideally recommend you returning to the area you worked last. I had been a Community Staff Nurse and I was very hopeful they would find a placement back within this setting. Unfortunately, this was not possible and therefore my options were discussed for alternatives.

Your interview will probably focus on what type of practice placement aligns best with your previous nursing experience and the practicalities of managing the course commitments. However, it is likely that you will also be asked some values-based questions, so it is a good idea to think through some potential answers. Values-based interviews are designed to explore how a person might behave or think in certain situations. In nursing, of course, key professional values include compassion and empathy, honesty and a desire to learn. Questions may be framed to encourage you to explain what nursing means to you and what you have learnt during your break in practice. You may also be presented with hypothetical scenarios such as what would you do if a patient complained about an aspect of care you have provided, or how would you support a new member of staff. In preparing such questions course teams often consult with patients whose service user perspective brings valuable insight to the process. The following are extracts taken from written pre-interview responses kindly contributed by one of our previous students.

1. *What has made you want to return to practice now?*

   After leaving mental health nursing to care for my family, I initially started voluntary work which led to roles working with young children. I enjoyed the caring nature of this experience, but it made me realise how much I miss being able to practise previous nursing skills. Studying a CACHE (Council for Awards in Care, Health and Education) level 3 in Early Years confirmed my passion for and previous knowledge of mental health. This is the direction I would like to take in the long term, as I consider nursing a solid profession with excellent professional and personal development opportunities. My family situation is now more settled, and my children are older and less dependent. Therefore, shift work is realistic and bank nursing is an option I would like to explore as this may provide work flexibility around family life. I feel encouraged by campaigns to raise mental health awareness and government plans for much needed investment in mental health services.

2. *What qualities, skills or experience can you bring back into nursing following your break in practice?*

   After qualifying in 1998 I was able to build up knowledge from many years of experience in mental health nursing. My break in practice has confirmed my personal attributes of commitment, compassion for others, patience, and motivation to learn. My level 3 study in early years enabled me to revise social learning and attachment theories. This has given me a greater understanding of adults with mental health difficulties as well as broadening my knowledge of children's mental health. I feel I am naturally empathetic and have continued to apply the communication skills learnt as an RMN to my work outside of nursing. The experience of working with teachers, parents and families has enabled me to develop greater flexibility and increased my understanding of partnership working. Spending time as a full-time parent has given me another perspective on life and enriched my views on caring for others.

3. *What challenges do you think you will face during the course, and how do you plan to meet them?*

Being able to produce work at level 6 is likely to be a challenge, especially as my pre-registration training was not academic based. However, although I have completed a qualification at level 3 only, this has enabled me to plan study around family and work commitments. It also gave me experience of meeting deadlines and deepened my understanding of published research in areas such as brain development. I am a little anxious about how confident I would feel in placement which I know could be a pressurised environment with possible short staffing. My previous experience was mainly in community settings, so I have little ward experience and have not carried out basic nursing skills for some time. However, I am flexible and appreciate the choice of placement will depend on need and availability.

4. *What do you think you will find rewarding in returning to the nursing workforce?*

After time away I am really looking forward to hands on nursing care and being able to confidently resume practising as an RMN. It will be rewarding to bring together previous experience with new learning about current concepts in mental health. I hope to become more confident with physical health nursing skills and welcome the opportunity of working in an environment where there is encouragement to learn from the expertise of others. I feel the greater job security will enable me to plan career development and explore areas of nursing I had not previously considered. I feel the COVID-19 situation has raised the profile of nursing and confirmed to me the sense of meaningfulness a career in nursing can bring.

NUMERACY

As you will be aware competence in numeracy is a prerequisite for safe patient care. In daily nursing practice calculations are used in a range of tasks including medication administration, assessing body mass index, and measuring fluid balance. Working out drug dosages and infusion rates will vary according to the level of acuity of the area. With many medicines now Dossett-boxed or single unit-dosed, it could be argued that there is a risk of nurses in clinical practice becoming deskilled because this reliance on technology means they do not have to work out calculations daily. In some ways too, the dependence on calculators, whilst saving time, has also undermined our ability to carry out mental arithmetic. Nonetheless, and perhaps even more importantly, nurses have a responsibility to practise and retain their numeracy skills. Unfortunately, whether instilled during early education or simply a skill lost due to lack of practice, maths anxiety exists for many and is a well-recognised barrier leading to a lack of confidence with numbers. It has been described as an anxiety or tension that impairs performance (Ashcraft and Kirk 2001). Practice is the most effective way of overcoming this issue and regaining confidence. There are a wide range of free on-line resources to guide you in building competence and accuracy. Depending on your level of knowledge you can start with very basic calculations and gradually progress to the more complex. There will also be opportunities to reinforce this learning in the clinical setting.

As part of acceptance for a course place or to complete a Return to Practice course successfully, you will be required to pass a basic numeracy test. The questions are usually a mix of simple arithmetic and calculations based on balancing fluid charts and drug dosages. There are usually practice papers available which will give you some insight as to the type of questions. Preparation and practice are key to refreshing this skill and feeling confident. In the box below we have included some examples to give you an idea of what to expect.

Numeracy formulae and worked examples

General formula for calculating the number of tablets required per dose

$$Number\ required\ per\ dose = \frac{Amount\ prescribed}{Amount\ in\ each\ tablet/capsule}$$

General formula for calculating the number of tablets required per prescription

Number required per dose $\times$ *doses per day* $\times$ *number of days to be supplied*

Worked Examples

1. *500 mg is prescribed: the tablets are 250 mg. How many do you need per dose?*

   Applying the formula: $\frac{500}{250} = 2$

   So, the answer is 2 tablets.

2. *1.2 g is prescribed: the available tablets are 150 mg. How many do you need per dose?*

   Applying the formula: 1.2 g = 1,200 mg: so, $\frac{1,200}{150} = 8$

   The answer is 8 tablets.

Calculating drug dosages based on body weight or surface area

Sometimes the dose is calculated based on a patient's body weight (mg/kg) or surface area (mg/m^2). This particularly applies to cytotoxic drugs, topical preparations and prescribing for children.

General formula for calculating the dose based on weight

Total dose required = dose/kg × patient's weight

General formula for calculating the dose based on surface area

Total dose required = dose/m^2 × body surface area

Worked example

Dose = 1.2 mg/kg. Patient's weight = 67 kg

1.2 × 67 = 80.4
The answer is 80 mg (once rounded down).

Percentages

Percentages are a common way of expressing a proportion of something and are useful for comparing different quantities. Percent (%) means 'part in a hundred'. Some drugs are expressed as percentages and so this means grams per 100 ml. So, 0.9% saline (sodium bicarbonate) has 0.9 g of sodium bicarbonate in every 100 ml (= 0.9 × 10 per litres = 9 g/litre).

General formula for calculating the percentage of a given quantity

$$\frac{What\ you've\ got}{100} \times percentage\ required$$

General formula for calculating what percentage one quantity is of another

$$\frac{Smaller\ number}{Larger\ number} \times 100$$

Worked example

How much is 42% of 775?
Applying the formula

$$\frac{775}{100} \times 42 = 325.5$$

So, the answer is 325.5.

If you are feeling anxious about the thought of maths and drug calculations, we would recommend that you take some preparatory steps prior to commencing your return to practice. There are a range of quick online maths and numeracy courses available. Some of our students have found these reassuring and helpful in refreshing skills. In addition, universities may be able to provide ongoing assistance for numeracy difficulties through one-to-one tutorial support.

Words of Wisdom

During the couple of years before I considered returning, I had enrolled onto a maths Adult Learning course mainly to rebuild my confidence as I hadn't used the maths that would be required of me for some time. Although I am still not the most confident in maths it certainly gave me the boost I needed to apply to the course.

NMC PROFESSIONAL STANDARDS

The underpinning contemporary professional frameworks governing nursing are the Nursing and Midwifery Council's Future Nurse: Standards of Proficiency for Registered Nurses (NMC 2018a) and Realising Professionalism (2018b, 2018c, 2018d). At the time of writing this book, those governing SCPHN are the Standards of proficiency for Specialist Community Public Health Nurses (2004); however, these have been updated in July 2022 and there may be some changes as SCPHN programmes are revalidated (NMC 2022). These standards are central to nurse education as they focus on the knowledge, skills and attributes pre-registered students need to achieve prior to gaining entry on to the professional register. Each educational establishment running NMC approved programmes are regulated and approved according to these standards.

Realising Professionalism is divided into three parts which collectively contain the proficiencies that specify the knowledge and skills registered nurses must demonstrate when caring for people of all ages across all care settings.

- Part 1 *Standards framework for Nursing and Midwifery Education* (NMC 2018b)
- Part 2 *Standards for Student Supervision and Assessment* (NMC 2018c)
- Part 3 *Standards for Pre-registration Nursing Programmes* (NMC 2018d) which includes *Standards for Return to Practice Programmes* (NMC 2019)

Returning to Your Nursing Field

The Future Nurse standards of proficiency (NMC 2018a) were devised following consultation with the professions and public to determine the type of skills and competency required of a nurse to practise safely and effectively in contemporary healthcare.

These are featured as 'platforms' and 'annexes', encapsulating the proficiencies, communication and relationship management skills and nursing procedures that constitute the role of the modern nurse. We will come back to these seven platforms and two annexes in Chapter 4, but we introduce them here and hope that for many of you the language will feel familiar and offer some reassurance:

Seven platforms

- Being an accountable professional
- Promoting health and preventing ill health
- Assessing needs and planning care
- Providing and evaluating care
- Leading and managing nursing care and working in teams
- Improving safety and quality of care
- Coordinating care

Annexe A

Communication and relationship management skills

Annexe B

Nursing procedures

NMC Future Nurse Standards (2018)

These standards of proficiency for registered nurses focus on preparing nurses for caring in diverse settings and across all life phases (NMC 2018). The health of the population is prominent with renewed emphasis on health promotion and preventing ill health. This may once have been the chief remit of practice nurses, school nurses and health visitors; however, now the expectation is that all nurses have a part to play in promoting health regardless of their background or the setting. Nursing as a profession needs to be able to offer person-centred care that is safe and compassionate across the lifespan. We have now an increasingly aging population, a greater incidence of long-term chronic conditions and complex co-morbidities coupled with the wide-ranging impact of preventable conditions from unhealthy lifestyle choices. The nursing workforce needs to be prepared and adaptable. Some of you may feel apprehensive about returning to a role that seems to have undergone so much change. However, a closer look will affirm that supporting the mental and physical health of patients, families and communities has always been central to nursing work. Very often health promotion advice occurs opportunistically and unexpectedly, illustrating the importance of Making Every Contact Count (MECC) – an enduring initiative set by Health Education England in 2011. The following sections are from an account written by a returner who was able to help a patient towards an improved quality of life.

Returner's Account

I wondered how I could gain relevant health promotion experience within a palliative care environment. My view of health promotion was encouraging people to make healthy lifestyle choices such as smoking cessation to prevent disease. Around the time I completed my initial nurse training, terminally ill patients tended to be omitted from health promotion discussions (Kellehear 1999). Richardson (2002) identified that healthcare professionals holding this 'traditional' view of health promotion may find it difficult to see the relevance to palliative care. However, the World Health Organisation defines health as a holistic term encompassing physical, mental and social well-being, and describes health promotion interventions as those designed 'to benefit and protect individual people's health and quality of life' (WHO 1978 and 2016). The overall aim of palliative care is to enhance quality of life (Stevens 2020: in Lister et al. 2020) and to enable individuals with life-limiting illness to be as well and as active as possible. McMurray (2003) reasons that palliative care itself is a health-promoting activity.

My patient (Mr. B) was a 78-year-old man with metastatic small cell lung cancer, admitted for symptom control. He had previously received radiotherapy and chemotherapy for his cancer and recently had become increasingly unsteady on his feet due to double vision and fatigue. He was also suffering from nausea and loss of appetite. I talked to Mr. B about what he hoped to get from his stay on the unit, and he expressed his wish to gain his appetite back and enjoy eating food again. He stated that even when he felt like eating, the food did not taste particularly good anymore. During our conversation, I noticed that his lips were dry and cracked and on further questioning Mr. B said his tongue was also sore.

Throughout the admission process, I used a conversational style of questioning to encourage Mr. B to voice his wishes and current concerns. My plan of care involved explaining the importance of oral hygiene to Mr. B. However, I noticed that he was becoming tired. I felt that this was not the best time to have an in-depth discussion. Instead, I briefly explained how improving his oral hygiene could help with some of his symptoms and left an information leaflet for him to read through at his own pace. Providing written information on a subject is one way of avoiding information overload (Ali 2017).

The following day I talked Mr. B through his mouth care regime which included twice daily brushing with a soft toothbrush, using a chlorhexidine mouthwash and artificial saliva gel regularly along with the antifungal medication he had been prescribed (HEE 2016). Mr. B now realised his deteriorating oral health may be impacting on his enjoyment of food and his appetite and he could choose to make this aspect of self-care a priority. However, he expressed concerns that due to his fatigue he sometimes lacked the energy to complete effective mouth care and sometimes forgot to do it. From listening to Mr. B, I was aware that it was important for him to retain as much independence as possible, so I suggested that the healthcare team would remind him about his mouthcare and would ask if he required any assistance. We would also ensure that the necessary equipment was close to hand if he wanted to do it himself.

Using effective communication strategies such as open questioning, listening and written methods (Ali 2018; Indra 2018), I was able to understand Mr. B's needs and empower him to develop the skills and understanding he required to promote better oral health which would, hopefully, lead to an improvement in his quality of life. By the end of his two-week stay in the hospice, Mr. B had shown a noticeable improvement in his oral health, his appetite had started to increase, and he was enjoying a selection of small meals.

Note: References cited in this account are to be found in the reference list at the end of the chapter.

What is important to remember is that as an RTP student you are returning to the register not undertaking a three-year programme to gain professional registration. This returning nurse is able to build rapport, using the empathy and listening skills she has finely tuned over years of practice. Like her, you too will have gained a range of skills and experience as a qualified nurse in your post-registration career.

The Future Nurse proficiencies may appear broad and diverse reflecting the motivation that nursing as a profession should strive to achieve a very high standard of clinical skills and knowledge. The objective is that newly qualified nurses have completed the theory and skills necessary so that they can transition to skilled practitioners after registration (Council of Deans 2016a). The outcome statements apply across all four fields of nursing. For example, a learning disability nurse will need to achieve proficiencies in areas such as sepsis; an adult nurse will need to understand the principles of play therapy; a children and young people's nurse will need to be cognisant in the signs of dementia; and a mental health nurse will have to demonstrate knowledge of wound management.

You may feel that your background is specific to a particular area and this new vision of nursing across all fields is overwhelming. However, it is understood and recognised that returners have expertise in their chosen field, and this is valued and needed. So, we have a balance between stretching at times to meet proficiencies intended to shape and build a future nurse who can command a range of proficiencies and skills to meet the needs of the 21st century and ensuring that experienced nurse returners can reclaim and further develop their own specialist practice. There may be those of you who have not worked after gaining registration and may feel very nervous about attempting to return. Generally, nurses who have not worked within that immediate post-registration timeframe still retain nursing knowledge and skills. With good support they can quickly regain confidence and competence and successfully reactivate their nursing registration.

RTP nurse students have one generic practice assessment document but also one field-specific placement. There is recognition in terms of the depth and breadth of knowledge and skills required to meet specific needs in their chosen or intended area of practice. The proficiencies within the assessment document accord with the requirements of the NMC (2018) Standards of Proficiency for Registered Nurses but with provisos for 'scope of practice' and 'intended field of practice'. These are pivotal terms for returning to practice which we will revisit in more detail in Chapter 4.

COURSE CONTENT AND STRUCTURE

As you might expect, most Return to Practice courses comprise theory and practice. An initial induction period is designed to familiarise you with higher education resources and processes and prepare you for your practice placement. A mix of topics will help you to refresh your nursing knowledge, reacquainting you with the Nursing and Midwifery Code and areas such as the use of clinical judgement, evidence-based practice and managing challenging behaviour. There may be opportunities to refine skills in mental health first aid, end-of-life care and health promotion. Importantly, induction will also include mandatory skills training such as basic life support, the management and administration of medicines, infection control and safe patient handling. Whilst most clinical skills are updated in the practice placement, provision is also made for workshops and skills simulation. Sessions will also address the use of library and online resources and advice about job seeking.

Courses vary in structure. Most will frontload information in the first few weeks, but many will bring students back together for further study days throughout the course. This encourages a paced approach and reinforces the benefits of peer support. If the course includes academic assessment, these later sessions will often focus on study skills, tutorials and assignment preparation.

Alongside face-to-face sessions, most courses will also use a distance-learning approach. This can be extremely helpful for those out of region students who would otherwise have long journeys to make. Studying at home will involve access to learning platforms. These are online spaces which contain all the necessary information and content required to undertake the course. Therefore, it is crucial to prepare by ensuring that you have a suitable digital device and reliable Wi-Fi connections. It is best to use a laptop or desk computer. Phones may work as a temporary stopgap, but their screen formats do not enable comfortable reading and can make some platform areas difficult to navigate. Broadly, online course content is usually delivered in two different ways. The first takes the form of a virtual lecture or seminar which happens 'synchronously' or in real time, facilitating live discussion and group work. The second is 'asynchronous' which refers to the use of online study resources undertaken independently in your own time. If all this online activity makes you feel anxious, please be reassured that it is simpler than it sounds, and support is always on hand.

The business of refreshing and updating knowledge and skills tends to straddle a broad base yet also cater for the individual needs of field-specific students. Generic topics such as reflective practice, team-working and leadership are likely to be addressed in a way that enables full cohort engagement and the exchange of different perspectives. However, timetables will also make provision for students to follow their own study path, whether that be health visiting or mental health nursing. Course teams include field lecturers who will provide specialist or field-specific sessions and individualised academic support.

PLANNING YOUR PRACTICE PLACEMENT

The choice of placement is usually made in discussion with student, course team and placement providers. To maintain consistency of support and assessment, students are generally allocated to one clinical area for the duration of the programme. The first guiding principle, therefore, is to return to a known area of nursing. Going back into clinical environments after time away can be demanding and anxiety-provoking. Indeed, venturing into a completely new type of practice setting can be too over-whelming and is generally not advised. Retaining some familiarity is both sensible and reassuring as this returner experienced.

Words of Wisdom

I am returning to adult nursing after a nine-year break. Prior to my break I spent most of my career working in a community setting. My placement area is a rural GP practice with a practice population of approximately 6,500 patients. I have worked at the practice for the last two years as a dispenser. A Practice Nurse post became vacant, and I felt that this would be an ideal opportunity to return to my nursing career. I decided to approach the surgery to see if they would support me whilst I undertook my return to practice module which they did. I will be working as a Practice Nurse in the surgery once I have successfully completed the course.

Of course, there are exceptions. Some students have a wealth of nursing experience and may have some choice as to which kind of placement is preferred. There are others who have little or no registered nursing practice to which to return. In this instance, a conversation may be needed with the individual to establish career aspirations and ensure that the course is the best option; sometimes, a period working as a healthcare assistant can provide the best platform from which to then apply to return to registered practice.

A second guiding principle is to prioritise the retrieval of acute nursing skills. This is especially pertinent for those who have been out of practice for a considerable time, or for those who have worked in healthcare roles that have taken them away from direct patient care. Updating in a fast-paced inpatient area can boost confidence and set the scene for return to nursing even if the subsequent nursing posts are less acute. Again, though, this approach is not for everyone. If you have always been a community-based nurse and want to return to this role, it makes little sense to opt for a hospital placement. Your expertise will be in primary care and therefore that should be the focus for your practice placement. Within the one setting, however, students are required to engage in a variety of practice learning opportunities to meet the required NMC RTP proficiencies and understand care for a diverse range of people.

The third guiding principle is to think through your ongoing nursing career. Practice placement providers are also workforce recruiters whose interest is in retaining returning nurses once they have completed the course. Very often, confirmation of placement necessarily involves the intention to accept employment following re-registration. Wherever possible, therefore, it is important to align this practice setting with your future plans. If you are a hospice nurse who desires to return to this area, an adult surgical ward placement is of little value. However, at a later stage following both placement and employment in the hospice sector, you may think again, perhaps choosing to change your career path with a move to an acute hospital environment. Once acclimatised to registered practice, it is quite common for returning nurses to move around until they find their natural fit.

Some placement areas can offer contractual arrangements so that the student can progress on to registered nurse employment in the same practice setting following successful course completion. In this instance, the return to practice process can encapsulate both course and job interviews effectively involving employer representatives and course teams. Successful applicants receive a salary (usually healthcare assistant pay scale) whilst in their supernumerary student role and can benefit from the sense of permanence and belonging which this arrangement affords. This route does however involve additional practice hours with a full- time commitment and therefore may not suit all individuals.

SUPERVISED PRACTICE HOURS

Most courses require returning nurses to undertake a minimum of 150 supervised practice hours and a maximum of 450 supervised practice hours within the course duration. You will have supernumerary status and will be able to arrange with Practice Assessors and Practice Supervisors (more on these roles in Chapter 4) as to when you complete these hours in the clinical setting. Whilst courses are designed to offer flexibility, it is important that practice hours coincide with the main activity of the placement and the working hours of assessors and supervisors. In most instances, this will entail completing mainly full shifts or days. With the Practice Assessor's agreement, it may be acceptable to work occasional shorter shifts. However, it is important to recognise that achievement of proficiencies cannot be assessed if practice has not been observed over the full range of a working day.

As a minimum, you will need to prepare to be in placement twice a week. Some students find it easier to front load the placement hours because this quick immersion in practice provides them with continuity, speeding up retrieval of confidence and competence. They may finish their placement early, allowing time to work on any required academic course components. Others may prefer a more paced approach, undertaking two to three shifts a week over a more sustained timeframe. Once you have established a pattern that works for you, small variations can be added in – for example, you may attend placement for three to four days before taking a week's holiday. Course durations can be extended slightly, but generally need to be completed within the six-month limit. Reasons for this are multifaceted and include the need for a formal structure within which progress can be monitored and evaluated with action planning put in place if appropriate. Also, each placement has varying capacity to support and assess students dependent on numbers of supervisors and assessors available at any given time.

SPECIALIST COMMUNITY PUBLIC HEALTH NURSING (SCPHN)

SCPHN practitioners consist of health visitors, school nurses and occupational health nurses. They operate from two active NMC registrations – nursing or midwifery and specialist community public health nursing. SCPHN Part 3 of the register builds on the original nursing or midwifery qualification. Therefore, returning SCPHN practitioners who have lapsed both registrations will need to address both sets of practice proficiencies. This presents a particular set of challenges and is one of the reasons why Return to Practice courses for this smaller group of practitioners are less widely available. Course providers are listed on the NMC website with contact details for further information. Even if the nearest course is some distance away, it is still worth making inquiries with your local NHS Trust; some placement providers work with universities to support students through their return to practice, having already interviewed them to fill potential vacancies following successful course completion. In this instance returners may receive a negotiated salary whilst in their supernumerary student role. Care is needed to ensure that job and student roles are clearly delineated so that students have the time and space to retrieve knowledge, skills and confidence. However, this employment route can be a good option, offering greater job security and a chance to get to know the team. If your SCPHN registration rests on a midwifery registration, it is likely that you will need to complete two consecutive RTP courses. Even if this is not the case, some Return to Practice courses require SCPHN returners to complete two placements (one for nursing and one for health visiting). Others have amalgamated the two in one primary care setting where the core placement is centred on health visiting but with opportunities built-in for students to work with a nursing team and be assessed by a nurse Practice Assessor. Those who have maintained their nursing or midwifery registration only need to complete the SCPHN Return to Practice route.

Currently, the V100 (prescribing) is also updated once the programme proficiencies are achieved, and registration reactivated. However, new SCPHN standards have just been published (NMC 2022) triggering changes to the way RTP courses for SCPHN are likely to be run over the coming years.

Returning SCPHN practitioners are required to undertake between 150–450 supervised practice hours within the 4–6 months course duration. These hours are titrated according to individual needs and time out of practice. The following table is used as a guide by placement providers when calculating the number of practice hours for each SCPHN returner. Student status is supernumerary and practice hours can be negotiated with assessors. Even though transferable skills exist and are recognised in nursing and SCPHN practice, the course will feel like a full-time commitment for many students. Normal course duration for SCPHN students is therefore flexible to accommodate the required hours and individual needs but must be completed within a maximum of six months from commencement.

Years out of practice	Minimum practice hours required	Equivalent days in practice(7.5 h per day)
5–10 years	150 hours	20 days
11–20 years	300 hours	40 days

Source: Abbott, S. et al., 2012 / City University London / Public Domain.

MIDWIFERY

Some universities also offer a pathway to return to midwifery. This matches nursing and SCPHN routes and may also be completed via the Test of Competence or the traditional approach via a supported supervised practice placement. The application process and benefits are very similar with funding and stipend payments in place. Again, too, some organisations will work in conjunction with course providers, offering an employment arrangement (often as a healthcare assistant) whilst supporting you to return to the clinical setting. This offers some advantages providing a gentle way back into contemporary practice. Skills and academic knowledge can be updated in a diverse range of practice environments supported by experienced midwives, and with the advantage of some financial provision whilst undertaking the course. Every course is slightly different, so it is important to make individual inquiries.

PREPARATORY STUDY AND READING

Words of Wisdom

Before applying, I signed up for an online subscription to the *Nursing Times* to at least have some more up-to-date information and to help my understanding of more current issues.

From initial inquiry to confirmation of a course place there is likely to be a period of several weeks or months. So, what is it that a returning student should be reading? A good place to start is with the nursing press. Journals such as the *Nursing Times* and *Nursing Standard* are accessible online and will give you a quick summary of current issues. You may also want to refresh some basic anatomy and physiology relevant to your area of practice. Apart from a nursing dictionary, we would encourage you to resist the urge to buy textbooks as this can be expensive and may result in random purchases which turn out not to be particularly useful. The Health Education England (HEE) website offers helpful information regarding returning to practice. The NMC and Royal College of Nursing websites are also useful with a wealth of resources regarding current nursing and health-related topics.

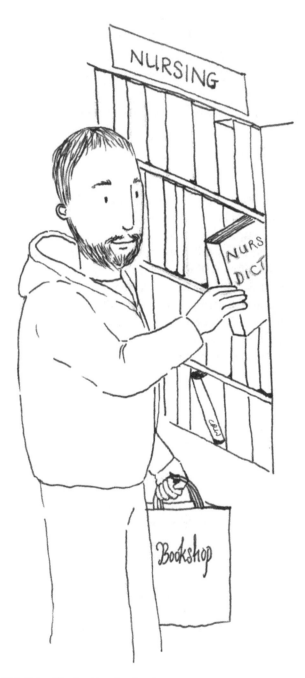

ILLUSTRATION NO. 2.1   Student buying book.

ARE YOU READY?

Before you apply for a Return to Practice course ensure that you have enlisted the support of those around you. As already discussed, assistance can come in all shapes and sizes. Talk to your family, friends and even neighbours if appropriate and accept all offers! Courses are usually part time, but the reality will often feel more like full time. This is especially true when you are completing your practice placement and towards the end when you are likely to be working on your academic assignments. Course teams wish every applicant to be successful; however, they also need to be assured that you have thought through the implications of undertaking this challenging return journey. At interview you will be asked about what support networks you have in place, so it is vital to have a firm plan. If at this point you realise that you are not quite ready, it may be wise to defer your application to a later course intake. We have known many to take their time. A little like a long jumper poised to run and leap through the air, it is not unusual for returners to prepare and even apply, but then pause and not go forward until the moment feels right.

REFERENCES

Abbott, S., Anto-Awuakye, S., Bryar, R., and Trivedi, S.G. (2012). Returning to health visiting practice: completing the circle. *Community Practitioner* 85 (9): 25–29.

Ali, M. (2017). Communication skills 2: overcoming the barriers to effective communication. *Nursing Times* 114 (1): 40–42.

Ali, M. (2018). Communication skills 5: effective listening and observation skills. *Nursing Times* 114 (4): 56–57.

Ashcraft, M.H. and Kirk, E.P. (2001). The relationships among working memory, math anxiety, and performance. *Journal of Experimental Psychology: General* 130: 224–237.

Cambridge English Dictionary (2022). Available at: https://dictionary.cambridge.org/dictionary/english/assumption.

City University London (2011). Return to Health Visitor Practice Guidance Notes.

Council of Deans (2016a). https://councilofdeans.org.uk/wp-content/uploads/2016/08/Educating-the-Future-Nurse-FINAL-1.pdf.

Creary, S.J. and Gordon, J.R. (2016). Role conflict, role overload, and role strain. In: *The Wiley Blackwell Encyclopedia of Family Studies* (ed. C.L. Shehan). John Wiley & Sons Inc.

Health Education England (2011). Making Every Contact Count (MECC).

Health Education England (2014). Nursing return to practice: review of the current landscape.

Health Education England (HEE) (2016). Mouth care matters: a guide for hospital health care professionals. Available at: https://mouthcarematters.hee.nhs.uk/2016/12/01/mouth-care-matters-guide-hospital-healthcare-professionals

Indra, V. (2018). Effective communication skills for nursing practice: a review. *International Journal of Nursing Education and Research* 6 (3): 311.

Kellehear, A. (1999). *Health-Promoting Palliative Care*. Oxford: Oxford University Press.

McMurray, V. (2003). Health promotion in palliative care. *Cancer nursing practice* 2 (9): 35–39.

NMC (2016). Social media guidance. https://www.nmc.org.uk/globalassets/sitedocuments/nmc-publications/social-media-guidance.pdf.

NMC (Nursing & Midwifery Council) (2018). *The Code. Professional Standards of Practice and Behaviour for Nurses, Midwives, and Nursing Associates*. London: Nursing & Midwifery Council.

NMC (2018a). *Future Nurse: Standards of Proficiency for Registered Nurses*. London: NMC.

NMC (2018b). *Standards for Education*. London: NMC.

NMC (2018c). *Future Nurse: Standards of Proficiency for Registered Nurses*. London: NMC.

NMC (2018d). Realising professionalism: standards for education and training. Part 2: standards for student supervision and assessment. 2018c. https://tinyurl.com/y7kfynub.

NMC (2019). *Realising Professionalism: Standards for Education and Training*. Part 3: Standards for return to practice programmes. London: NMC.

NMC (2022). SCPHN standards https://www.nmc.org.uk/globalassets/sitedocuments/standards/post-reg-standards/nmc_standards_of_proficiency_for_specialist_community_public_health_nurses_scphn.pdf.

Nursing and Midwifery Council (2004). *Standards of Proficiency for Specialist Community Public Health Nurses*. London: NMC.

Richardson, J. (2002). Health promotion in palliative care: the patients' perception of therapeutic interaction with the palliative nurse in the primary care setting. *Journal of advanced nursing* 40 (4): 432–440.

Stevens, A.M. (2020). Symptom control and care towards the end of life. In: *The Royal Marsden Manual of Clinical Nursing Procedures*, 10e (ed. S. Lister, J. Hofland and H. Grafton). Oxford: Wiley & Sons.

World Health Organisation (1978). International conference on primary health care. Declaration of Alma-Ata. *WHO Chronicle* 32 (11): 428–430.

WHO (2016). Health Promotion. WHO [online] Available at: https://www.who.int/news-room/q-a-detail/health-promotion

USEFUL WEBSITE

British Dyslexia Association https://www.bdadyslexia.org.uk.

CHAPTER 3

Bridging the Gap

Returning to practice is about closing a gap in time. Whether you have been away from the profession for four years or twenty years, the sense of what you no longer know and what you can no longer do may feel quite uncomfortable. Gaps in knowledge and practice will need to be scaled, but you will be coming back with new insights and skills which you may not have possessed before. Understanding these gaps through a process of self-assessment and support from others will help you to focus not so much on what you have missed, but rather on what is ahead. Once you start to engage with practice and study, your way forward will become clearer.

This chapter will focus on the self as a learner and as a returning nurse. Your journey back to nursing is one of transition from one self-identity to another. In the previous chapter we suggested that a review of your current roles and commitments is good way of preparing for this change. A return to a former identity – nurse – brings with it both reward and responsibility. Where much needs to be achieved in a relatively short space of time, knowledge of self can arguably be the most significant determinant of success.

SHARING HOPES AND FEARS

At interview, you will be asked why you wish to come back to the profession. You may need to explain your preparation for the course, your future goals and your current situation. There may also be a question about your hopes and fears. Articulating your personal challenges and aspirations to others enables you to hear them out loud too, and this is important in defining the way ahead. Listening to the hopes and fears of other returning nurses should also affirm that you are not alone. As already mentioned, the opportunity for peer support is one of the most beneficial aspects of Return to Practice courses. There will be formal and informal occasions where you will be able to exchange thoughts and feelings with other students. Some of your hopes will find common ground with others, and many of your fears will be shared. Speaking out your anxieties in a supportive environment can be immensely helpful both in terms of affording reassurance, and in acknowledging individual strengths. You may be the most computer-literate person in the class but have been the longest out of practice; consequently, you will have skills to share and advice to receive.

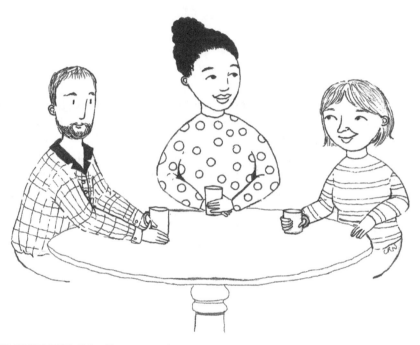

ILLUSTRATION NO. 3.1   Peer support.

Hopes	Fears
I will still love nursing as I used to	I will find the nursing role has changed so much that I can no longer relate to it
I will pass the course	I will struggle to complete the academic assignments
I will manage to juggle all my commitments	I will find it difficult to complete all the course requirements on time
I will find a job	I will not be successful in finding a job
Practice teams will be understanding of my role as an RTP student	In practice there will not be the time and space I need to regain my confidence and competence
The Practice Assessor will be friendly and supportive	I will not get on with my Practice Assessor

THE GAP

At the start of the journey most returning nurses feel acutely aware of the gap in time between now and when they last nursed. Whatever the actual number of years in question – and this can vary enormously – the perception of something wide and scary is experienced by many students. As soon as applicants come together, we try to disarm this fear by asking them to share with each other their number of years out of nursing. This helps promote reassurance and a sense of companionship. In truth, we have found that a successful return to the profession does not seem to correlate with the length of time away, and this is also borne out in Coates and Macfadyen's qualitative study (2021) where, despite initial anxieties, students concluded that they were able to retrieve competence irrespective of the nature of their gap in clinical practice.

Words of Wisdom

I was particularly worried about how long I had been out of nursing practice. I had a gap of about 11 years. This felt an extremely long time and although I was confident in basic nursing skills, I was aware other areas may take more time to relearn. However, that is one of the differences with the return to practice in that you are relearning skills rather than learning them from scratch. Both course tutors were very reassuring about this length of time not being a problem in returning to nursing.

There are of course a range of steps which can be taken by those who feel an interim stage is advisable. Some returners lead up to the course by first working as a Healthcare Assistant or volunteer; indeed, some are already support workers, then discovered to be nurses and strongly encouraged by their colleagues to apply to return to practice.

Most returning nurses face the prospect of going back to the healthcare environment with a mixture of apprehension and excitement. Your gap in practice will have been filled with other valuable life experiences which will equip you with a maturity and insight for nursing of which you may not be fully aware. Many a third-year student or newly qualified registrant has been quick to perceive and access the rich reserves of experience and compassionate knowing that lie just below the surface of the nurse returner; and many returners have felt the sudden boost in confidence that comes when their skills and understanding are sought in this way. Such a day often marks a turning point.

Similarly, you may also feel worried about the thought of studying again. Adult learners can experience higher levels of anxiety and self-doubt than students who enter higher education straight from school or college (Navarre Cleary 2012). Often our experience of learning is based on previous experiences, and these can impact either positively or negatively. You may feel that you have little to bring to the table in the classroom situation. When undertaking academic development, key factors inhibiting progression for adult learners can include lack of confidence in ability and fear of failure (Quinn and Hughes 2007). This can be the reality for many mature students, and are common fears cited by nurses returning to practice.

Anxieties may be related to practice or study, or both! However, it is important to remember that often the easiest way to learn is to start by recalling what you already know. Part of the experience of returning to practice is about adapting and applying previously gained knowledge and skills. This, of course, takes time.

Words of Wisdom

The placement progressed, and I grew in confidence as my skills improved. Interestingly, I noticed that the combination of the life skills I had acquired during my time away from nursing plus my renewed clinical expertise gave me a resilience I had not had before. Managing complex situations did not seem quite so challenging.

After an initial lack of confidence, this returner has started to feel empowered. The challenges remain, but now she perceives her life experience transform into a new resilience. This is self-efficacy.

SELF-EFFICACY – A HELPFUL CONCEPT

Self-efficacy is concerned with how we think, feel, behave and become motivated to succeed despite difficulties (Bandura 1997). When we achieve something, we feel enhanced by a strong sense of self-efficacy and improved personal well-being. Goals and aims are viewed as challenges to be attained rather than personal threats to be avoided. It is useful here to break down the expression to further understand the concept. 'Self' is the identity of a person, and 'efficacy' is simply a more formal way to say effectiveness. It is derived from the Latin verb 'efficere' which means to work out or accomplish (Oxford Dictionary 2017). Self-efficacy therefore enables us both to effect and feel achievement. It is a conscious awareness of a personal ability to be effective and control actions (Zulkosky 2009). Bandura (1994) explains that the defining attributes of self-efficacy may be viewed as intrinsic to the learning process. We perceive the capability to do something; the confidence to do it – the 'I can do' – and, most importantly, the perseverance to pursue the doing of it despite challenges along the way. Taylor and Reyes (2012) suggest that self-efficacy plays a major role in behaviour and motivation impacting on all areas of our personal and professional lives.

Returners are faced with the gap in knowledge and skills that exists between now and when they last practised. They must believe that this gap can be bridged. To make this happen, they must trust that they will be able to retrieve and update what they once knew. Our self-belief influences the choices and decisions we make based on the skills we believe we possess. When we have lower sense of self-efficacy, we limit our experiences and tend to stay within a comfort zone. Self-efficacy is the personal judgement of how well one can perform and achieve. It is situational, task dependent and impacted by several dynamics. Once goals are achieved this can encourage a higher sense of self- efficacy and prompt us to take on additional goals and more complex situations. Each achievement boosts your sense of confidence in your ability to achieve.

Thus, self-efficacy is a continuous and affirming process, yet nonetheless at times difficult to sustain. The reality is that there are differences in what we can and cannot do. Multitasking at home will not feel akin to managing the care of a group of patients – at least, not at first. Walking back into a healthcare setting may spark a fear of risk or failure which can be paralysing. It is important, therefore, to acknowledge that these first steps may be slow, setting small realistic goals which are achievable and so instilling confidence in the ability to progress. Bandura (1977) outlines four principles of self-efficacy which may provide a useful template for returning nurses.

Vicarious Experience

We learn from others. Observing those around us accomplish their goals can be inspiring. If we see others achieve success this encourages us to think, 'Yes, I can do it too!' At the start of you practice placement it can be helpful to seek out a role model who accords with your personal values and provides insight into the contemporary nursing role.

Verbal Persuasion

Encouragement is a big motivator. When those whose views we respect persuade us of our potential, we feel strengthened to make the effort to succeed. Constructive feedback from assessors, supervisors and tutors can reassure and re-energise, illuminating the way ahead. This can be particularly helpful midway through a practice placement when there are still challenges ahead to tackle, and the finish line is not yet in sight. Close friends and family members will also spur you on – these people are often very invested in your success.

Mastery Experience

This refers to past successes. Previous experience of overcoming obstacles and being able to do something well builds self-belief. As once registered and practising nurses, you know what it means to have the skills and knowledge to do the job, and therefore this is something that can be achieved again. Sharing information about your nursing history with other people in the team will reinforce a sense of earlier achievements.

Psychological Response

Thinking positively is a choice. Some placement days will be hard going; some of your academic work may fall below your usual standards. The overall picture, though, is likely to be of a busy person making steady progress towards re-entry to the nursing workforce. This is the achievement which matters. How we respond to situations is influenced by our psychology. Striving to maintain a positive outlook and minimising stress as much as possible will make the journey more enjoyable and promote self-efficacy.

Well known for her enduring study skills publications, Cottrell also points to the importance of managing your experience as a student (Cottrell 2019). She enthuses that higher education has the potential to be transformational, stretching students to achieve self-efficacy, providing a view of future success and encouraging a thirst for knowledge. Cottrell is referring to three-year undergraduate study, but she could be talking about Return to Practice. For all its short duration, a sense of surprise and self-revelation often accompanies course completion.

Words of Wisdom

I have learnt that I like myself!
I actually do want to go back to work and to health visiting.
I was more able to manage change than I previously believed.
It's surprising how much you are capable of.
Make it your own learning – get what you want from it.
I know more than I thought I did.
Do not fear change!
I have discovered that I enjoy studying and learning.
I need to have more confidence in myself.
It feels like a massive achievement!
I am looking forward to further study.

CONFIDENCE AND COMPETENCE

If we could only use one word to sum up returning to practice, that word would be 'confidence'. The journey for nearly all returners is one of regaining confidence. Be reassured that you do have a rich resource of experiential knowledge on which to draw; however, nervousness and anxiety are part of the process. Although you may initially feel like a fish out of water, you will find your stride and your confidence, and competence will follow close behind.

Here is what many returners have told us over the years:

Words of Wisdom

I felt a lack of confidence in returning to practice.
It was a reminder of the skills I already had but had forgotten that I had them! You do know more than you think you do – your skills are still there and relevant.
I realised my knowledge gap was not as big as I thought it was – I did not feel lost.
Combatting personal anxieties about the placement was challenging.
Returning to the practice setting and realising that I have skills which I haven't been using was a good and almost immediate feeling.
I was surprised how much nursing knowledge and skills I have still retained.
There were moments when I realised that I knew more than my mentor!
It was nice to be asked things by other students.
I still know things! I haven't lost all my skills!
Regaining my confidence in practice took time.
Can I do it? I can do it.

The journey to reclaim and reaffirm nursing knowledge and skills will have its highs and lows. Confidence and competence come together but in small steps. As your past nursing experience comes to the fore you should feel more emboldened to move forward. However, uplift in confidence happens differently for individuals. Some returners feel an immediate relief when they commence practice because none of it is as difficult as they thought it would be. Others report this progression as more of gradual upward curve. For some, a run of consecutive shifts enabling continuity and validation through team involvement heralds a key turning point. With regaining confidence comes that sense of returning to something known and feeling valued. As returners make this reconnection, most are reminded of how much they have missed nursing.

Words of Wisdom

I really felt that I was back where I belonged.
It felt like I was coming home.
Being in placement felt right – I've found where I belong.
Both placement and hospital were enthusiastic and encouraging – I was made to feel very welcome.

SELF-ASSESSMENT

Gaps in practice and study may be felt acutely but be hard to visualise. However, grappling with the nature of their form and shape will help you to understand something of the journey ahead. Priorities need to be identified and objectives established; and therefore, it is necessary to engage in self-assessment. This can be a challenging and complex activity. Many of us shy away from the thought of having to pin down our strengths and weaknesses. There is often a tendency to be over-critical of ourselves, and this can negatively skew our self-belief. Even with self-confidence and strong commitment, it can still be unclear as to how to put these positive energies to good use. Transferable skills may be highly valuable but perceiving them can be problematic (Hughes-Morris and Roberts 2017). In their study of SCPHN courses where qualified nurses return to full-time student status, Hughes-Morris and Roberts found that, as mature and established professionals, SCPHN students needed to feel that their existing skills were respected before they felt open to new learning. Coates and Macfadyen (2021) came to similar conclusions on polling Return to Practice students about their experiences back in the clinical setting. Supernumerary status was welcomed by many as a protective cloak allowing time for orientation and observation. However, it was the sharing and acknowledgement of prior nursing knowledge and experience that proved to be most significant factor in helping returners to regain confidence and competence.

Self-assessment may feel awkward and tricky, but it does ensure a balanced picture where individual strengths must be noted alongside areas for development. Lifelong learning is intrinsic to our professional career as registered nurses, and assessment of self is a major part of that ongoing pursuit. Most believe it to be a skill which benefits from practice and guidance from others. To that end, we have included here two examples of a self-assessment process, the first completed by a returning learning disabilities nurse and the second by a returning health visitor. We hope you find them helpful.

RTP student self-assessment and development tool: Nursing
This self-assessment is a prior learning check that is designed to help you to identify what skills and expertise you currently have. At the same time, it will inform on areas where study or clinical skills and knowledge may need developing. There are three sections – prior experience, prior study and scope of practice. Please complete this self-assessment in preparation for your practice learning experience, taking into consideration your prior learning and experience in relation to the standards of proficiency (Nursing and Midwifery Council (NMC) 2018), course outcomes and their intended scope of practice upon readmission to the NMC register.

Section 1: Prior experience	
Nursing	*Learning disabilities – primarily with autistic children and adults.*
Healthcare-related	*Cared for my elderly parents in recent years.*
Other	*I have worked as a teaching assistant for special needs. I was also a first-aid instructor.*

Areas for future development

To retrieve and develop proficiency and knowledge in learning disabilities after being out of practice for twelve years.

To regain confidence and competent in team working and co-ordinating and refresh my leadership skills.

To gain competency in the administration of medications within the clinical area developing my knowledge of policies and procedures used within the setting.

Section 2: Prior study	
I can use or have access to a computer	*I have basic skills including accessing the internet, using email and word processing.*
I have experience using digital tools	*No – not at all.*
I can search for and access journals and articles	*I have done this in the past but will need an update.*
I can write an academic essay	*I have retained some skills, but do not feel confident about academic writing. I am hoping it will come back as I start to practise it again.*
I can use literature to reference my work	*Yes, I know how to do this, but welcome a refresher.*
I can critique articles and books	*I can critique; however, I am not confident about this skill.*
I understand the use of reflective practice	*I have written reflective accounts before, but I would need support. I have found this skill quite challenging.*
Do you have any additional learning needs that we need to be aware of?	**Yes** ☒ **No** ☐ Dyslexia

(continued)

(continued)

> **If you have answered 'yes' to the above question, please discuss with the Course Leader.**
>
> *Please can you outline any support/adjustments that are currently in place or any support adjustments that you have received in a previous learning environment. Student Support plans can be put in place to support you in your learning.*

RTP student self-assessment and development tool	
Section 3: Scope of practice (Nursing – all four fields)	

Please review your scope of practice in the light of your prior experience, knowledge and skills. The NMC expect return to practice students to refresh or develop skills specific to their chosen area of practice. **At pre-placement stage you may not be fully aware of those areas you need to identify; however, thinking through areas of strength and areas for development can be helpful in preparing you for your early discussions with your Practice Assessor and Practice Supervisors.**

NMC Future Nurse Standards: 7 platforms	Self-assessment
1. Being an accountable professional	*Understand basic values of confidentiality, trust, compassion and being professional. Need to re-acquaint with NMC Code.*
2. Promoting health and preventing ill health	*Interested and contribute to supporting public health. Recent role as first-aid instructor means I have confidence about basic health promotion and first responses.*
3. Assessing needs and planning care	*Still able to assess basic needs and plan care due to recent care of family members. Will need to update.*
4. Providing and evaluating care	*Able to assist others with personal hygiene and basic needs such as hydration, nutrition, etc. Will need to refresh skills beyond this level.*

5. Leading and managing nursing care and working in teams	*Past nursing roles have encompassed leading and managing others. Have not been in leadership role for some years and so will need to build up confidence.*
6. Improving safety and quality of care	*Aware of basic mechanisms such as audits and patient feedback but feel very rusty knowledge-wise.*
7. Co-ordinating care	*Have worked as nurse co-ordinator in the past, but not confident now as so much has changed since I last nursed.*
Annexe A: Communication and Relationship Management Skills	
Underpinning communication skills	*I feel I have good communication skills which should be apparent once my confidence has returned.*
Communication skills for supporting people to manage their health and prevent ill health	*Yes, quite good in this area due to recent role as first aider and instructor.*
Communication skills for therapeutic intervention	*Yes, I need to regain specific knowledge, but I feel I can communicate therapeutically.*
Communication skills for working in professional teams	*Not so confident here.*
Annexe B: Nursing Procedures	
Care and support with rest, sleep, comfort and the maintenance of dignity	*Aware of importance of rest and sleep. Understand and have worked to maintain the dignity of others.*
Care and support with hygiene and the maintenance of skin integrity	*As a carer I have recent experience of caring for skin integrity and ensuring that pressure areas are monitored.*

(continued)

(continued)

Care and support with nutrition and hydration	*Past nursing experience included the care of PEG feeding and ensuring fluid balance. Have worked with assessment tools and used them widely with clients with learning disabilities to support their health and understanding of dietary advice.*
Care and support with elimination	*Experience in supporting others with elimination needs. Have helped individuals towards self-care. Some experience with colostomy care but need to refresh these skills and knowledge.*
Care and support with mobility and safety	*Have looked after both elderly and young clients with a broad range of mobility issues. Also have some experience in liaising with occupational and physical therapists.*
Care for respiratory care and support	*Basic skills and understanding only. I will require support and supervision to update in this area.*
Support with the prevention and management of infection	*Have supported others to understand infection risks and prevention. Understand the principles of aseptic technique although do not have wide experience in this area. Will need to focus on this aspect.*
Care and support at the end of life	*Some experience in caring for individuals at end of life. However, not confident in this area.*
Medicines administration	*I have not administered medicines for a long time, so this would be a priority focus.*

Please note that new NMC SCPHN standards were published in 2022; however, at the time of writing the 2004 SCPHN standards are still approved for use for RTP courses and are sufficient here to provide a basis for self-assessment.

RTP student self-assessment and development tool: SCPHN
This self-assessment is a prior learning check that is designed to help you to identify what skills and expertise you currently have. At the same time, it will inform on areas where study or clinical skills and knowledge may need developing. There are three sections – prior experience, prior study and scope of practice.   Please complete this self-assessment in preparation for your practice learning experience, taking into consideration your prior learning and experience in relation to the standards of SCPHN standards of proficiency (NMC 2004*), course learning outcomes and your intended SCPHN practice upon successful readmission to the NMC register.

Section 1: Prior experience	
SCPHN	*Four years of Health Visiting and nurse prescribing. Health promotion and working with vulnerable families.*
Healthcare-related	*Background in general nursing with a focus on surgical settings and stroke rehabilitation. During break in practice have worked as agency support worker in community settings.*
Other	*I have worked for a range of charities including the Stroke Association UK and Epilepsy Society. I have a master's degree in Advanced Healthcare Practice.*
Areas for future development	
Update knowledge on Prescribing and current recommended products *Current protocols around health visiting and child protection*	
I can search for and access journals and articles	*Utilised online library journal searches but would need support with searching for journals in the library.*
I can write an academic essay	*Previous experience writing academic essays for my Master's, although this was some time ago.*
I can use literature to reference my work	*Used referencing before I just need to learn Harvard technique.*
I can critique articles and books	*Yes, I have previous experience.*

(continued)

(continued)

I understand the use of reflective practice	*Regularly reflect on all things that I do. I have used several different models in the past.*
Do you have any additional learning needs that we need to be aware of?	Yes ☐ No ☒

If you have answered 'yes' to the above question, please discuss with the Course Leader.

Please can you outline any support/adjustments that are currently in place or any support adjustments that you have received in a previous learning environment. Student Support plans can be put in place to support you in your learning.

RTP Student self-assessment and development tool

Section 3: Scope of practice (SCPHN)

Please review your scope of practice in the light of your prior experience, knowledge and skills. The NMC expect return to practice students to refresh or develop skills specific to their chosen area of practice. **At pre-placement stage you may not be fully aware of those areas you need to identify; however, thinking through areas of strength and areas for development can be helpful in preparing you for your early discussions with your Practice Assessor and Practice Supervisors.**

NMC Standards of proficiency SCPHN (2004): Principles of public health practice	Self-assessment
Collaborative working for health and well-being.	*I have worked closely with MDT members including physio, OT and speech and language teams. I do need to familiarise myself with the MDTs that I am going to be involved with as a health visitor.*
Working with, and for, communities to improve health and well-being	*Previous HV experience providing information/ education to facilitate informed decisions about health and well-being. I need to update my knowledge in this area.*

Developing health programmes and services and reducing inequalities	*I need to update within the health visiting role.*
Policy and strategy development and implementation to improve health and well-being	*This is an area that I will need to work on.*
Research and development to improve health and well-being	*I have not been an active researcher. I am aware of the requirements for evidence-based best practice and need to re-discover current best practice for health visiting.*
Promoting and protecting the population's health and well-being	*I am an active listener and I feel that I have ability to effectively support others.*
Developing quality and risk management within an evaluative culture	*I will need to update my knowledge in this area.*
Strategic leadership for health and well-being.	*I have had experience effectively communicating within teams and leading in some areas.*
Ethically managing self, people and resources to improve health and well-being.	*I feel that I work well and ethically.*

A recent evaluation of this new self-assessment process drew a positive response from the cohort. The students acknowledged that it had felt daunting to complete the tool so early in the course. However, they also reported that having to articulate their past skills and achievements to others had proved to be a focusing experience, helping them to re-affirm their nursing identity and status within practice placement teams.

THE LANGUAGE OF NURSING

In the early days of the return journey just retrieving the language of nursing can be challenging. Language enables us to orientate, understand and navigate the world around us. It helps determine our nationality and our culture, and within these broad parameters it also binds us into professional and social groups where we develop what Higgs et al. term 'a fine-grained subcultural identity' (2004, p. 57). Professions communicate their values using specialised language which includes terms and abbreviations known only to those inside the organisation.

Language underpins all our nursing interactions and is crucial to patient outcomes and safety. As you will remember, communication regarding patients must be succinct, relevant, and current, and it needs to convey universal meaning to all nurses. However, there is still no common language that reflects all that we do as nurses, embracing both the complexity and diversity of our patients' conditions and the care we plan, give and document. So, although we pride ourselves as effective communicators, this is open to interpretation. The nursing role is often one of co-ordinator shifting constantly between professional teams and members of the public. Nurses generally communicate in an ordinary language so that patients can understand, but they have a short code for each other, and a different specialist terminology for their allied healthcare colleagues. Consequently, messages can become lost or misread.

Current processes for documentation via computerised records may underpin our practice and address accountability and liability; however, they have no capacity to record shorthand phrases such as 'watch that heel' or 'push fluids' understood at nursing handovers. Therefore, it is important to avoid misunderstandings and be clear and aware of the significance of the expressions we use. Electronic health records are fast becoming a reality and the drive for a standardised nursing language is also gaining momentum as it facilitates fluent communication between multi-professional teams and improves quality of care (Rutherford 2008).

Naturally, over the years the language of nursing has evolved. Terminology can change from Trust to Trust and region to region so there may be some differences that you will need to adapt to in the clinical setting. Despite being frowned upon, abbreviations persist and are commonly used in patient documentation. Various specialties have developed their own language which can cause confusion and lead to misinterpretation by others not in the same field. CPD for a midwife means Cephalopelvic Disproportion and signifies the potential for a difficult labour that may require intervention. CPD in another context refers to Continuous Professional Development – something entirely different, and without the same impact! Another mystery to unpack comes in the form of DAT: Diet as Tolerated or Drug Abuse Testing? Date of Admission (versus Dead on Arrival) is also a more pleasant outcome. All are in use. We also recall one European nurse returner who was told to unlock the CD cupboard; expecting to find a stack of music recordings, she was shocked to find instead shelves of controlled drugs. Most areas now have an agreed list of abbreviations for use within the setting with strict guidance in place to avoid ambiguities and their potential impact on patient safety.

This lack of standardisation has received long-standing criticism not just in the UK but also globally. Some progress has taken place in the area, but there is more to do (McLachlan et al. 2020). Perhaps some of these problems are understandable. Nursing sits astride many disciplines, borrowing terms from medicine, biology, business and the social sciences. This is exemplified when we look at the range of words that we have for those in our care: are they patients, clients or service users? It is likely that we would all answer differently. It can be an emotive question for returning nurses because it speaks to what you hold dear – your remembered values and your time in nursing.

WHAT HAS BEEN HAPPENING WHILST YOU HAVE BEEN AWAY?

Healthcare will have changed since you were last in the clinical setting. That does not mean that there have been great advancements and movements in all areas. In some respects, little has altered. However, a brief review of our recent history may shed light on some of the contours in the landscape. It may also bring back into focus your own nursing journey including your starting and stepping off points.

Nurse education has undergone numerous changes, evolving from hands on training (including a two-year course to gain an enrolled status or three years for registration) to Project 2000 which stipulated a minimum diploma level, but advocated a degree level and so moved nurse education into universities. The drive to increase the status of nursing as an all-graduate profession was constant and evidenced in degree programmes for nurses in larger cities throughout the UK from the early 1970s; ultimately, this became mandatory in England in 2013. You will have your thoughts about what kind of educational route works best, and the topic often sparks animated discussion for returners as each defends or critiques their own nurse training. Although this 'old school' versus 'graduate profession' argument is likely to fade over time, it may always elicit some interesting and useful discourse.

As you will be aware nursing students became supernumerary in 2005 which meant they were not included in the workforce. Since the 1980s, due to the European Union framework, the minimum hours and the topics covered for nurse education were standardised in line with regulations to facilitate freedom of travel and work. The hours were set at 4,600 with at least 50% in the clinical setting. Various Higher Educational Institutes (HEIs) have autonomy in terms of hours, provided minimum requirements as stipulated by the NMC are met. However, this has resulted in variations in levels of exposure and experience gained by students throughout their pre-registration programme (Eaton 2012).

To meet the needs of an increasingly changing and diverse population, the future role of the nurse is envisioned as one of technical and clinical speciality standing astride all four nursing fields (NMC 2018b). Several strategies have underpinned this ethos including Modernising Nursing Careers (DH 2006), Preceptorship Frameworks (2010) and the Willis Commissions (2012, 2015) – all of which provide useful context and background. The Future Nurse standards (NMC 2018b) verify the crucial role played by the nursing profession in the implementation of this vision for the NHS and they are aligned with its aims. It was recognised that nurse education should focus further on developing leadership and management skills, interprofessional working and political awareness to increase the scope of knowledge needed in caring for people across lifespans in diverse settings. With an increased range of skills and proficiencies to be achieved across a wider domain of practice, the changes propose to make 'top of licence' practice the aspiring model for nurse registration. For some returners, this future vision may have a familiar ring, chiming with their own experience of training which facilitated clinical learning at the bedside.

Some further changes in healthcare provision to note have issued from the NHS five-year-forward review which has seen a shifting focus of care from acute settings to primary care (NHS England 2014). With greater longevity comes an increase in complex long-term conditions and so this movement out of hospitals and into the community makes economic sense. Inpatient beds have decreased by 50% in the past thirty years according to the Kings Fund (2021); this means that patient turnover is greater with advances in medical science and technology allowing for more complex procedures in a much shorter timeframe. The NHS Long Term Plan (NHS England 2019) moves forward with Integrated Care Systems which involve different approaches such as allowing people to have more control over service provision in their area with closer collaboration between GPs and community services. General practice and community nurses are at the forefront of meeting the needs of the population acting as ambassadors for health promotion and an enhanced quality of life. They are generally lone workers with a broad range of skills which help them to remain flexible and adaptable in often challenging situations. To address the ever-widening gap in health inequalities, improvements in health promotion and access to support services are planned. The aim of the Future Nurse Standards (NMC 2018b) is to equip nurses to work in any setting at the point of registration. Consequently, pre-registered students are spending more time in primary care and community placements, learning how to apply their knowledge and skills in a range of diverse environments. Return to Practice placements within community services are feasible. However, due to the specific skills required, it is recommended that returners have some prior experience of these roles to help facilitate an easier transition.

PROFESSIONAL VALUES

We know, of course, that good nursing practice is underpinned by robust professional values. The mid Staffordshire NHS Trust inquiry served sadly to damage the image of caring competent professionals, highlighting appalling breaches in care and professional judgement. This crisis levelled scrutiny and criticism at nursing as a profession (Francis 2013a). Following the Francis report recommendations, Willis was commissioned with a clear mandate to review the state of nursing education for possible inadequacies which may have ill-prepared nurses for contemporary practice (Willis 2015). Initial concern had triggered views in the media that a graduate route for nurse education was placing too great a focus on academic skills to the detriment of traditional caring values. However, no major issues were identified; in fact, Willis was reassuring, documenting that nurse graduates were competent and significant players in the drive for quality outcomes in patient healthcare (Willis 2015). Ultimate conclusions concurred that poor skill mix and low staffing/patient ratios have the biggest impact on quality of care and patient safety (Currie et al. 2005; Hayter 2013).

Nonetheless, the impact of the mid Staffordshire public inquiry was far-reaching. In 2012 the Chief Nursing Officer at the Department of Health adopted a new strategy encompassing six core values which reflected quality-driven effective care. The 6 Cs within the framework (shown in Figure 3.1) embrace moral values, professionalism and dedication and remain fundamental to today's nursing care.

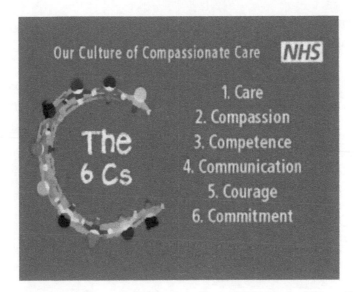

FIGURE 3.1 NHS Culture of Compassionate Care. *Source:* NHS England/Open Government Licence v3.0.

In 2015 the NMC added an additional C to address the honesty due to patients and families when things do not go as they should. This is a duty of 'Candour' which, like all the core values, was encompassed within The Code (NMC 2015) and updated in 2022 (NMC 2022). This was enhanced in 2016 with a further strategy called Leading Change, Adding Value, which introduced ten commitments placing emphasis on leadership and partnership working, public health and the use of research and technology (NHS England 2016). In conjunction with the 7 Cs, these are paramount in establishing and supporting therapeutic relationships and fostering consistency in quality of care provided.

As returners you may be familiar with some of these strategies, or you will recognise the core principles that underpin practice. Our professional values are captured under the themes of the NMC Code which is updated every few years to ensure that contemporary nursing can respond to the needs of a changing world. As you take the next step back into practice and into a role underscored by a chief instruction to protect the public, one piece of advice from past returners shines out like a beacon: know the Code.

Words of Wisdom

As I progressed through the placement, I realised I wasn't expected to know about every medical condition or get bogged down by reading up on everything! Learning the NMC Code and concentrating on the 'Standards of proficiency for registered nurses' was at the core of what I needed to know, for the placement, the course and for the future. So, I would recommend becoming very familiar with them and do keep going back to them to focus your learning.

Prioritise people: Practice effectively: Preserve safety : Promote trust:

Personal professional responsibility

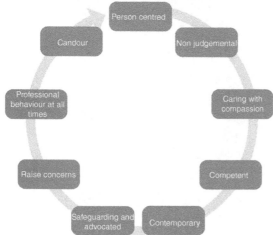

Employer organisation responsibility
- Access
- Choice
- Safe staffing ratios
- Resources
- Transparent
- Good Leadership
- Quality assurance
- Supportive learning environment
- No blame culture

FIGURE 3.2   NMC Code.

The current Code encapsulates four themes which reflect the high standard of practice expected of nurses, regardless of student or registrant status (NMC 2018a). Founded on ethical principles of autonomy, beneficence, non-maleficence and justice, the Code keeps our practice safe ensuring that we support the rights of the individual, sustain the well-being of others, cause no harm and maintain respect and fairness (Beauchamp and Childress 2019). In this respect, the Code becomes a trusted guide. The themes are listed below, with Figure 3.2 best portraying how they correspond to responsibilities at individual and organisational levels.

- Prioritise people
- Practice effectively
- Preserve safety
- Promote professionalism and trust

Here is a summary of key points to take forward as you prepare to leap across that gap!

- In the early days, take small steps and set achievable goals.
- Use a diagram to track your journey from one achievement to the next.
- Do not compare yourself with others; everyone is on a different journey.
- Keep a diary of your progress.
- Use resources to help you and enlist the support of peers and colleagues.
- Learn from feedback on how to move forward.
- Keep going. Failure is due to lack of knowledge not to lack of ability.
- Stay positive.

REFERENCES

Bandura, A. (1977). Self-efficacy: toward a unifying theory of behavioral change. *Psychological Review* 84: 191–215.

Bandura, A. (1994). Self-efficacy. In: *Encyclopedia of Human Behavior*, 4 (ed. V.S. Ramachaudran), 71–81. New York: Academic Press.

Bandura, A. (1997). *Self-efficacy: The Exercise of Control*. New York: Freeman.

Beauchamp, T.L. and Childress, J.F. (2019). *Principles of Biomedical Ethics*, 8e. Oxford University Press.

Coates, M. and Macfadyen, A. (2021). Student experiences of a return to practice programme: a qualitative study. *British Journal of Nursing* 30 (15): 900–908.

Cottrell, S. (2019). *The Study Skills Handbook*. Macmillan International. Red Globe Press.

Currie, V., Harvey, G., West, E. et al. (2005). Relationship between quality of care, staffing levels, skill mix and nurse autonomy. *Journal of Advanced Nursing* 51 (1): 73–82.

Department of Health (2006). Modernising nursing careers—setting the direction. http://tinyurl.com/2kux5o.

Department of Health (2010). *Preceptorship Framework for Newly Registered Nurses, Midwives and Allied Health Professionals*. London: Department of Health.

Eaton, A. (2012). *Pre-registration nurse education: a brief history* http://www.williscommission.org.uk.

Francis, R. (chair) (2013a). *Report of the Mid Staffordshire NHS Foundation Trust Public Inquiry*. The Stationery Office.

Hayter, M. (2013). The UK Francis report: the key messages for nursing. *Journal of Advanced Nursing* 69 (8): e1–e3.

Higgs, J., Richardson, B., and Abrandt Dahlgren, M. (2004). *Developing Practice Knowledge for Health Professionals*, 57. Butterworth Heinemann.

Hughes-Morris, D. and Roberts, D. (2017). Transition to SCPHN. *British Journal of School Nursing*. doi:10.12968/bjsn.2017.12.5.234.

The King's Fund (2021). NHS hospital bed numbers: past, present, future. www.kingsfund.org.uk/publications/nhs-hospital-bed-numbers.

McLachlan, S., Kyrimi, E., Dube, K. et al. (2020). Towards standardisation of evidence based clinical care process specifications. *Health Informatics Journal* 26 (4): 2512–2537.

Navarre Cleary, M. (2012). Anxiety and the newly returned adult student. *School for New Learning Faculty Publications*. 5-1-2012. Chicago: DePaul University.

NHS England (2014). NHS five year forward view. NHS England, London. www.england.nhs.uk/ourwork/futurenhs.

NHS England (2016). Leading change, adding value, a framework for nursing, midwifery and care staff. https://www.england.nhs.uk/wp-content/uploads/2016/05/nursing-framework.pdf.

NHS England (2019). *The NHS Long Term Plan*. NHS England.

NMC (2004) Standards of proficiency for specialist community public health nurses. NMC.

NMC (2018a). *The Code. Professional Standards of Practice and Behaviour for Nurses, Midwives and Nursing Associates*. NMC.

NMC (2018b). *Future Nurse: Standards of Proficiency for Registered Nurses*. NMC.

NMC (2022). The professional duty of candour. https://www.nmc.org.uk/standards/guidance/the-professional-duty-of-candour.

Nursing and Midwifery Council (2015). *The Code: Professional Standards of Practice and Behaviour for Nurses and Midwives*. London: NMC.

Nursing and Midwifery Council (NMC) 2018. Future Nurse: standards of proficiency for registered nurses. Available at:https://www.nmc.org.uk/standards/standards-fornurses/standards-of-proficiency-for-registered-nurses.

Oxford English Dictionary (OED) (2017). Oxford: Oxford University Press.

Quinn, F.M. and Hughes, S.J. (2007). *Quinn's Principles Practice of Nurse Education*. Cengage Learning.

Rutherford, M. (2008). Standardized nursing language: what does it mean for nursing practice? *The Online Journal of Issues in Nursing* 13 (1). http://www.nursingworld.org/OJIN (accessed on 31st May 2022).

Taylor, H. and Reyes, H. (2012). Self-efficacy and resilience in Baccalaureate nursing students. *International Journal of Nursing Education Scholarship* 9 (1).

Willis, P. (2012). Quality with compassion: the future of nursing education. Report of the.

Willis, P. (2015). Shape of caring: a review of the future education and training of regis.

Zulkosky, K. (2009). Self-efficacy: a concept analysis. *Nursing Forum* 44 (2): 93–102.

CHAPTER 4

Practice Placement

FIRST STEPS

You will have now completed your university course induction and met the rest of the cohort, sharing with them your hopes and fears about returning to nursing. You have refreshed your Basic Life Support skills, revised the principles of infection control and studied the most recent publication of the NMC Code. You have your uniform, and you have purchased some sensible comfy shoes. All you must do now is turn up for your first day. At this point, many of our previous students would chorus 'Don't panic!' They would also want to share memories of the anxieties they felt when walking on to placement that first time. Here is how one student expressed her feelings:

Words of Wisdom

Before I started my placement, I felt a myriad of emotions. Excitement and looking forward to the experience mainly, but also, I couldn't help feeling nervous and slightly overwhelmed by it all. How much was I expected to know? What were they expecting of me? Was I good enough to be in this position? How was I going to be received as an RTP student? On reflection, these were all normal fears and worries about starting somewhere new but as I had been out of nursing for ten years, when I put on that uniform for the first time, I felt like I could be out of my depth and couldn't help feeling I had imposter syndrome!

Returning to Nursing Practice: Confidence and Competence, First Edition. Ros Wray and Mary Kitson.
© 2023 John Wiley & Sons Ltd. Published 2023 by John Wiley & Sons Ltd.

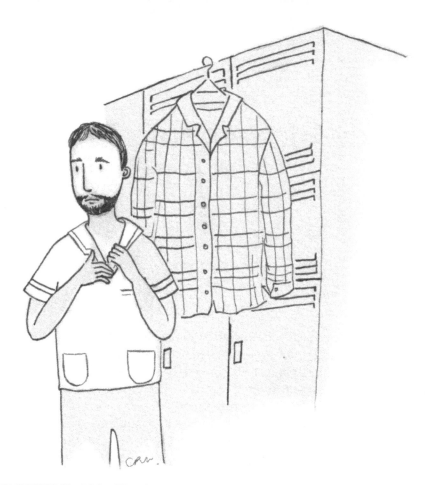

ILLUSTRATION NO. 4.1A   First day.

We can all remember the tentative steps taken at the beginning of our careers as we ventured into the unknown. The clinical setting is where pre-registration student nurses are cultured and moulded and hopefully where they blossom, and it is here too where your practice skills will be reawakened. Of course, first impressions are important and therefore engaging in some level of preparation will help you to establish a way forward and feel more in control. Early contact with an identified placement link person can ease anxiety and be reassuring. In addition, each placement or Trust will usually have a website which will provide a general overview of the area.

Shown in Figure 4.1, Maslow's hierarchy of needs (1987) suggests that basic physiological needs such as food, shelter and clothing are paramount before we can successfully progress to meeting higher order needs such as esteem and self-actualisation. Simple things such as travel routes to your placement and parking can cause untold stress if left until the last minute. Have a trial run a few days before so that you can navigate that difficult junction more smoothly and know where to park the car! Make sure that you pack food and drink – something sustaining and perhaps with a favourite snack that will help to mark the achievement of getting through this first day.

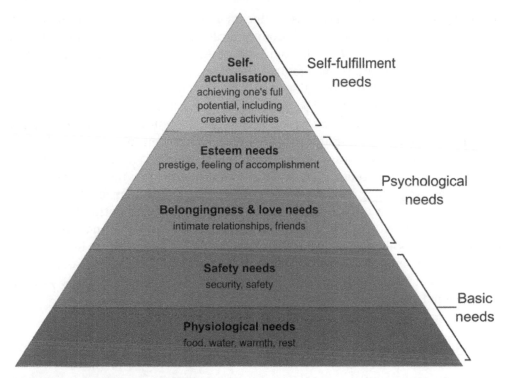

FIGURE 4.1 Maslow's theory (1987).

Once a basic level of physiological comfort is secured, Maslow encourages us to attend to our psychological needs, chief of which concerns the forging of positive relationships. Former students stress the importance of those first contacts with placement staff and advise returners to use their communication skills to build early rapport. A smile goes a long way even when you do not feel self-assured. Try to be open and friendly, interested and curious, yet not too needy. This is all common sense, of course, but, as we know, nerves can make us question even the most basic responses. The one thing you may feel sure about is what you do not know or cannot do. The evidence suggests that the gap in contemporary practice for returners is keenly felt (Morton-Cooper 1989; Coates and Macfadyen 2021).

It does help to remember your days as a staff nurse supporting students. Revised guidance from the NMC places quite a weight of responsibility on qualified nurses in terms of the levels of support, interaction and supervision they should provide to students, so it is likely that your supervisors and assessor may also feel apprehensive and under scrutiny. A pre-placement visit can serve many purposes, identifying shift patterns and rotas, initiating introductions and helping to ease that 'first day' feeling. Robinson et al. (2013) identified that anxiety has a major impact on cognitive processes, so it is important to alleviate this if you can. Tell them about yourself and your nursing background. Some nursing team members will be quite inexperienced so disclosing your nervousness may help them to share theirs. You may be surprised by their response! By the end of the placement many will have learnt from you, but at the beginning it is important to recognise your own individual needs as a learner and wait for your confidence to strengthen. Communicating and discussing your previous experience is crucial and will help your Practice Assessor and Supervisors to understand your starting point. We will return to Maslow later in the chapter when we take a more detailed look at the transition back into nursing practice.

Each returner's journey will be different. Everyone likes to be acknowledged and valued and, of course, you may have a wealth of experience. However, it may take some time to find your feet and reclaim your sense of identity and credibility as a nurse. For some, knowing that you will not be expected to be 'all singing and all dancing' will bring a sigh of relief. It will allow you time to settle into the new arena as you strive towards regaining confidence and competence. Others may feel slightly indignant or frustrated at loss of status; however, this learning opportunity should be viewed positively as student status offers a juncture to re-hone and develop new knowledge and skills. The period out of practice will vary between each individual but returning to an area of nursing which has some level of familiarity is reassuring and can help to restore confidence. The first small steps may be hesitant, and the road ahead seem daunting, but this is the start of your journey.

Words of Wisdom

Relax, you don't have to know the answers. You are there to learn. I didn't recognise the equipment used to take a patient temperature and had to ask how it worked before I could carry out this simple task. It may be challenging to feel such a novice, but keep in mind your ultimate goal. If you're mistaken for a qualified nurse politely remind the person you are training. If you feel intimidated by how out of date you feel or how much has changed, recall you don't need to tackle everything at once. You are bringing a whole wealth of past life experiences to this course. You can draw on these to remind yourself to break challenges down into bite-size pieces – which placement objectives are you trying to achieve today? Make time to acknowledge and celebrate your successes with your mentor as you recall nursing practices and learn new ones.

PRACTICE PROVIDER INDUCTION

At some point before you begin your placement or within the first few weeks, it is likely that you will receive an official introduction from your placement provider. Generally, each trust or organisation has an employee induction programme that you will be able to access as a student. Returners are welcomed and valued as potential workforce and, following course completion, are often recruited into registered nursing posts by their placement providers (Health Education England 2014). Induction programmes, therefore, are designed to generate a sense of belonging in the broader team and present an opportunity to make new friends. Practical information related to uniforms, ID badges, staff support, parking and security are usually addressed at these sessions. The following is not exhaustive but provides a list of other topics and areas usually covered either face-to-face or via e-learning:

- Orientation to Trust, department and role
- Conditions of employment
- Development and training
- Health and safety
- HR policy and procedures
- Personal development
- Nursing induction – Safe Patient Handling and Resuscitation
- Access to Trust IT systems including intranet

If you are undertaking an NHS placement you will be issued with an NHS Smartcard to access electronic data on clinical services. This will be unique to you and has an electronic security certificate. You will be assigned a PIN to unlock the card using a system very similar to the chip and PIN bank cards. The card allows healthcare professionals access to clinical and personal information related to patients, although the level of access does vary according to role. The smart card is used with a password and this information should not be shared as the access is secure and auditable. Each time access is requested a record is created so this information can be viewed to determine what the user was accessing and when. Patients' right to privacy means that they should be informed as to who and why their information is used and shared with other healthcare professionals. There is a duty of care to individuals to protect confidentiality related to health and care information so stringent application processes and security exist to protect these systems. If your placement is in the independent sector, you will find equivalent ID security systems in place. As well as a general welcome, one of the aims of practice provider inductions is to showcase the values and objectives of the organisation. This may lead you to ponder on where and how you will fit as a returning nurse.

FINDING YOUR FEET

Words of Wisdom

Patients are people first. Basic nursing care and humanity will never change. Yes, I was slow at washing patients to start with – so much so, the other staff asked where I had worked before! I didn't know where anything was or how to use the electronic medication management system, but I kept reminding myself that I had something to offer – an abundance of life skills – and I was a nurse once, even if it did feel like a lifetime ago.

At times contemporary practice may seem more complex and challenging, but it remains ever rooted in the fundamentals of basic human kindness. Many returners feel an almost immediate reconnection with patients, often unaware that their instinctive responses to the needs of others create a positive role model right from the start.

Words of Wisdom

Patients stay the same.
The opportunity to meet patients and be a positive influence in their lives is a joy.
It has been great meeting patients again and being with students.
The best thing has been the patient contact and feeling you have helped as a nurse.
Care doesn't change because people don't change.
I had forgotten how much I like patients and how great it is to receive thanks for giving care.
I have loved getting back to patient contact.
Being back with patients is very fulfilling.
I have enjoyed communicating with patients again.
I felt needed.

The sense of fulfilment at being back in touch with patients provides early affirmation for many students regarding their decision to return to nursing. However, there is a journey to travel and a transition to make. A degree of self-questioning is inevitable and normal at this stage, and for many there is an initial pain barrier (mild to moderate in most instances) to traverse. This discomfort can be eased by knowledge of what lies ahead. We would recommend that you familiarise yourself with your programme requirements and outcomes; this is unlikely to be needed on your first day, but if asked, it will help your confidence if you are conversant with this information.

Words of Wisdom

Read the course guides or module handbooks – they contain useful information.
Try to get a good understanding of the practice requirements, but don't feel too overwhelmed!
Understand the assessment and exactly what is required; give yourself time to settle into your placement but keep in mind the work that needs to be completed.
Try to get something completed early on.

'Transition occupies a space between what went before and what is evolving' (Benner 2010). These words preface work by a key social scientist and nurse theorist, Meleis, who researched the nature of transitions. She defines transition as a potentially stressful process occurring over time, characterised by phases, and often made more difficult by the weight of individual expectations (Meleis 2010, p. 41). In the early days of placement Return to Practice students describe their uncertainty about what others will expect of them and what they should expect of themselves. Benner's acclaimed work on levels of nursing proficiency (derived from the 1981 Dreyfus model of skill acquisition) may provide some guidance here (Benner 2005). Five transitional stages – novice, advanced beginner, competent, proficient and expert – show how nurses develop their nursing practice. We have summarised these stages below:

Novice

This first level represents new student nurses who have no previous experience of practice. They are unable to predict or plan patient care and need to rely on received instructions and basic rules. Their performance will be limited because they have little understanding of context and reality of practice settings and situations.

Advanced Beginner

This stage reflects the knowledge and skill level of newly qualified nurses who have some understanding of patient situations but little depth of experience. Even within a holistic approach, their focus is on completing tasks.

Competent

These are nurses with two or more years of registered experience. They are starting to be able to organise with efficiency but require a deliberate and conscious approach to planning. They can read patient situations accurately and have good management skills.

Proficient

At this level, nurses have speed and flexibility. They are increasingly able to predict situations (seeing them as whole events), recognising and responding to patterns of behaviour and understanding connections and adapting to change.

Expert

Expert nurses have 'an intuitive grasp of each situation' based on their deep knowledge and experience (Benner 2001, p. 32). Their actions are not based solely on rules, but on an understanding of what is needed and relevant at any given time.

The stages match the nursing journey from Year 1 student through to advanced nurse practitioner, so how can we usefully apply this model to your return to practice? A sense of which of Benner's stages you had reached before your break in practice may give some indication as to where you might reasonably expect to re-enter the profession and should also help to keep self-expectations realistic. It would, though, be simplistic and inaccurate to draw exact and direct parallels because the experience of returning to a once well-known practice is not the same as learning that practice for the first time. More usefully, however, Benner identifies three further aspects which run beneath these five stages. These offer a closer alignment. The first is a movement from a practice based on rule-following to one which draws on knowledge gained from previous experience. This is highly pertinent for returners who must at first seek out the new rules and facts required for contemporary nursing before they can reconnect with remembered patterns of knowing from past nursing roles. The second aspect concerns progression from needing to know all the components towards a sense of appreciation of the whole; again, returning nurses must fuse previous nursing experiences with the new reality. Finally, the third movement marks the shift from detached viewer to fully involved practitioner. These stages or movements are clearly perceptible in the following observations made by a Practice Assessor where we see the student moving from observer to questioner to practitioner.

Words of Wisdom from a Practice Assessor

During the placement my RTP student initially stuck to her supervisor and did not take initiative to complete tasks. She asked questions about procedures and linked to possible theories. As she became more confident, she was able to work more independently and rationalise easily which theory met her practice and why. She became more patient centred, was able to delegate and started putting herself forward for tasks such as coordinating and participating in MDT meetings.

Returners report that the transition back to registered practice is gradual. Initially, many ask to shadow nursing staff, preferring to observe and acclimatise before stepping into a more active role. This stage may feel very tentative and akin to pre-registration nurse training; however, as we have already stated, the returner role is very different. There is a hidden entity – 'the bit in the middle' – at first unexpressed and unknown, which represents your past nursing knowledge and experience, and which needs to surface (Coates and Macfadyen 2021). As we discussed in the previous chapter, engaging in self-assessment prior to practice can feel like stumbling around in the dark; however, once grasped, this activity can give direction and shape to your learning journey, helping to pave the way for later conversations. Once a returner can perceive, interpret and merge current practice with what they remember from before, role transformation is enabled. From then on, every week in the clinical setting marks forward movement, punctuated by moments of self-recognition as a sense of professional identity strengthens. What was perhaps less clear at the start of placement now becomes visible to assessors, supervisors and the wider team facilitating greater understanding and more specifically targeted support. By the end of the placement many returners are viewed more as colleagues than students, esteemed by their teams and valued for their contributions.

However, let us return to Maslow's hierarchy of needs as it provides a valuable framework to work with during this transition as a returner (Maslow and Lewis 1987). Although arguably simplistic and certainly generic, the stages are progressive with achievement of basic needs facilitating the meeting of higher needs. This provides a helpful visual representation to the transitional process of returning to practice where each week marks upward movement – hopefully!

Basic Physiological Needs: Security and Juggling

Words of Wisdom

The first few shifts were physically and mentally tiring. I considered what I needed to achieve and how I was going to do this. On my days off, I batch cooked and prepared frozen meals. I organised online food shops to be delivered and I let friends and family know that I would be concentrating on my placement.

Initially the sheer exhaustion was the worst feeling; I remember the course leaders telling us to ask any family or friends to do some jobs at home to help, and in hindsight I think this advice is worth taking.

Maslow's first level of needs underlines care of self and others. We have already stressed the importance of securing your physiological needs for breaks and sustenance at the start of your placement. Whilst Return to Practice programmes are flexible and student status is supernumerary, runs of shifts or days in practice can be physically and mentally exhausting. Accumulatively, long hours, busy clinical environments and, perhaps navigating an unfamiliar journey home, will take their toll. The impact on family life does need to be considered. There will be stresses and strains along the way particularly if you have other commitments such as family responsibilities.

Words of Wisdom

It was challenging to do placement, academic work and look after family at the same time.

Juggling childcare and family life was not easy.

Fitting the course in with outside commitments was difficult at times.

I was trying to juggle written work, practice placement, job and running a home and family.

The hardest thing was juggling other commitments and managing time.

I had to arrange childcare and 12-hour shifts, and then needed to be flexible to fit with mentor's shifts.

Many nurses reflect on the balancing of roles as the most challenging element in their return to practice journey. There are potentially many balls to keep in the air including childcare, study, part-time jobs, placement hours and household tasks. Good time management helps along with considering all offers of help. Ask yourself questions and try to be honest with your answers when it comes to everyday jobs. Do I really need to iron everything? Could someone else do the school run today? Do I have to create every meal from scratch? Often students remark that, far from causing chaos and disorder, a change in habits can enliven family life and enable others to step up. Breakthroughs have been reported resulting in surprise teenage accomplishments such as doing the washing or making beds! It is important though not to throw out activities which you find relaxing and enjoyable. Rest and time out with family and friends must be factored in as they are intrinsic to success.

Words of Wisdom

Be kind to yourself – breathe!
It can be tiring – take a break!
Keep fit and healthy!
Don't be too hard on yourself in placement – you are there to learn!
Think about your physical fitness – stretching; wear comfy shoes!
Throw yourself into the programme and ignore the housework!

Psychological Needs: Self-Esteem, Belongingness and Feeling Valued

Maslow's middle range needs reinforce the importance of forging relationships. Once basic needs are met, and the environment and team feel friendly and familiar, self-esteem will flourish. It is timely here to affirm that nurse returners are very much welcomed and valued by healthcare teams; your contributions are important. However, with nervous energies at their height and everything feeling awkward, few returning students experience a full sense of belonging right at the start of their placement. Practice settings are usually very busy and, of course, patients must always take priority. You may feel yourself driven by a state of hyper-alertness and struggle initially to know where to put yourself and how to be. This is normal and natural. You have re-entered an intense working environment and it can take time to find your footing and settle in. Pace yourself; keep your expectations at a realistic level; listen and observe; and try to come across as engaged and helpful, receptive and curious.

Words of Wisdom

Go into practice confidently – 'I am here to learn' – and go out of your way to get along.
Be mature and swot on the basic things.
Lower your self-expectations – at the start assessors and supervisors do not expect as much as you think.

> Make it your own learning; get what you want from it.
> Get bedded in...enjoy your placement!
> Go for it; you can do it; you will be supported, and everything will be explained.

Self-fulfilment Needs: Self-Actualisation and Professional Identity

Maslow's highest levels of needs are about attainment and realising future potential. Achievement is a gradual process, individual and relative, where each person's sense of self-fulfilment may depend on their rate of progression. With successful completion of the Return to Practice course and subsequent NMC re-registration comes the chance of self-actualisation situated at the pinnacle of Maslow's hierarchy of needs. Students share their feelings of pride and satisfaction along with aspirations to explore future career possibilities. In their Words of Wisdom, we hear a renewed sense of identity, which Coates and Macfadyen (2021) found to be one of the strongest themes to emerge from their study. Role and identity are key elements of the return to practice experience, and it is something that we come back to many times throughout the book.

Words of Wisdom

This is the best thing I have done for myself in a long time.
Returning to practice has given me back my identity.
I feel so proud of my achievement.
Finding myself again after years as a parent is a revelation.
I now feel part of a worthwhile and rewarding profession.
I made the right decision and I feel happier in myself.
I am getting my identity back to return to a job I enjoy.
I have rediscovered a part of myself that I didn't realise that I had lost.

TEAM WORKING

When we ask returners to describe what they have most cherished about their practice experience, many will speak enthusiastically about becoming part of a nursing team again. The prospect of what a team might expect of you as a returning student may feel daunting, yet also exciting. Returners are welcomed and acknowledged widely, especially by the nursing teams they join. Remember that you bring with you a fresh pair of eyes. As your confidence develops, you will be able to offer alternative perspectives, prompting debate and creative problem-solving. Whilst it may take time before you can perceive again the measure of your past knowledge and skills, a sense of camaraderie can come quite early into the placement. We have collated responses from cohorts over the last ten years, and this sense of joy at being back with fellow colleagues repeatedly echoes.

Words of Wisdom

I enjoyed being part of a team and having rapport with nursing colleagues
Being back amongst nurses and like-minded practitioners feels great.
It was great to feel part of a team again, working together and increasing my nursing knowledge and skills.
I felt respected and valued by the rest of the team.
The best thing about returning to practice was being valued as a team member because of my experience.
I felt that I was working with like-minded people again.
The feeling of being wanted and needed and part of a team was one of the most positive aspects of the placement.
People do value and respect your past nursing experience.
I began to realise that I had valuable experience to offer.
Working in friendly teams was great.
I have been treated not as a student but as a colleague working with other professionals.
I have enjoyed engaging with colleagues across the organisation about nursing and the realities of looking after people.

As we all know, effective teamwork does not just happen when a group of people work together. It takes a coordinated effort with respect, communication and commitment to a common purpose. It is essential that team members are clear about the goals to be achieved, and understand their roles, responsibilities, and boundaries. There needs to be a shared purpose, good skill mix and a supportive ethos. It is well established that effective teamwork promotes patient satisfaction and reduces staff stress and attrition (West et al. 2015). Historically the nursing team was small with various levels of responsibilities and autonomy. Nowadays, teams are more complex and made up of several healthcare practitioners. There are multidisciplinary teams (MDT) staff within a single setting, and multi-agency teams (MAT) which draw on staff across the broader health and social care organisation. The NMC Code (NMC 2018a) stipulates that we work collaboratively across boundaries, thus encompassing an interprofessional stance. Collaborative working has been defined by Thistlethwaite (2012) as working together to achieve a goal that would have been less possible if undertaken by a single profession. There is growing recognition of the need for shared knowledge. Ultimately, of course, patient safety is paramount and increasingly seen as linked to effective team working. Simple tools and strategies exist to help teams function and more recently there has been investment in team training within healthcare (Hughes et al. 2016).

Nonetheless, you will know from previous experience that teams do not always work well, and therefore you may have some trepidation about re-entering the arena. Each returner will have different team-working experiences. Some may feel a little overwhelmed at finding themselves in a well-established senior team that seems initially inaccessible, whilst others may slot more comfortably into a friendly team, but then perhaps feel less challenged.

Remember that teams are fluid – people come and go, and goals can shift and change. Through his well-known model of team development, Tuckman (1965) reminds us that teams are in constant cycle, moving through phases of forming, clashing (storming), resolving (norming) and achieving (performing). More recently, Myers (2013) points to the dynamics within teams, describing the unconscious psychological energies that can impact on a team's behaviour and performance.

There are numerous models focused on team dynamics with one of the earliest suggested by Lewin in 1947 when he described group dynamics as the roles and behaviours people take on when they work within a team and how these impact on other team members. Belbin's work on team roles offers additional perspectives which can give insight into the behaviour of individuals (Belbin 1981, 2006). It is also well worth reading Belbin to see if you can work out your own team strengths.

BELBIN'S TEAM ROLES

Action-oriented Roles	Shaper	Challenges the team to improve.
	Implementer	Puts ideas into action.
	Completer Finisher	Ensures thorough, timely completion.
People-oriented Roles	Coordinator	Acts as a chairperson.
	Team Worker	Encourages cooperation.
	Resource Investigator	Explores outside opportunities.
Thought-oriented Roles	Plant	Presents new ideas and approaches.
	Monitor-Evaluator	Analyses the options.
	Specialist	Provides specialised skills

Source: Adapted from Belbin Associates (2006).

Here are some key areas of focus to consider as you return to the nursing team.

Clarity of Roles

It is important to be clear about your student role. This will help avoid confusion and facilitate realistic expectations. You are likely to have a wealth of experience to offer and may naturally wonder – 'Who am I in the team?' 'Where do I sit in the team?' As a returner your position is very different from a pre-registered newly qualified nurse. Although clinical and technical skills may be unfamiliar, your status as a mature life-experienced nurse will give you advantages. Arriving at the point of retrieved professional identity is not without challenge. Many students experience role ambiguity along the way, and this can cause some anxiety and uncertainty. This is well recognised by universities who provide specific uniforms and ID badges to help to define boundaries and give some clarity to the role and status of the returning nurse. Returners have a valuable contribution to make and are often adept at using transferable knowledge and skills in the clinical setting. As all involved continue to work together, they come to recognise and translate the worth of prior nursing experiences within the context of contemporary practice (Coates and Macfadyen 2021).

Personal Commitment and a Shared Goal

In common with other healthcare practitioners, returning nurses are usually highly motivated to achieve their goals (HEE 2014). You have decided to re-enter your profession, have invested in the process, and feel a drive to succeed. Whilst your knowledge and skills may feel slightly rusty, you are a professionalised individual whose past experiences and transferable life skills will enable quick socialisation back into the organisation and its teams. Once re-registered, the maturity and breadth of skills common to returning nurses tend to enable them to move up into more senior roles quickly (Stevens 2014). Therefore, it is important to believe in yourself and nurture the self-efficacy (discussed in Chapter 3) that spurred you to start this journey.

Support

Teams are made up of personalities and voices, each of which need to be heard. There may be different opinions, but this mix of perspectives, knowledge and skills can enrich team working. As nurses we understand the importance of effective communication, emotional intelligence and shared decision making. These are key contributors to a successful team and this in turn helps make a heavy workload more manageable. As we have already stated, returners often move quickly to an active team role, marking an upward trajectory where their advice and opinions are regularly sought by others.

Words of Wisdom

I established relationships with team members – knowing I could ask for help was so important. One of the sisters was a dragon but I could see she was the same with everyone, so I decided not to take her manner personally. After I found my feet, I realised that I had knowledge I could share. By the time I left, some of the clinical support staff and younger staff nurses were asking me for support!

Communication

Nurses have been identified as an 'essential point of communication' between patients, families and the multidisciplinary team (Francis 2013). Effective communication between team members is the glue that will hold everyone together. Although it may be some time since you last interacted with such a diverse group of people, you will be more skilled in communication and situational awareness than you may realise. With continuously advancing technology, today's care can be so focused on machines and equipment that the patient can seem lost. You may well have trained in earlier days when holistic care was the forefront consideration, and you were encouraged to spend time getting to know your patients. Goleman (2020) presents us with a range of defining attributes for emotional intelligence, chief of which include self-awareness and empathy, active observing and listening, and the ability to make connections with others. These are soft skills that we acquire as we go through life. Once you have settled, these skills will shine out in busy clinical settings, noted and appreciated by others. Think not of what your team have to offer you but what you can offer them. You may even be able to influence better practice.

> ### Words of Wisdom
>
> I observed my supervisor negotiating and delivering terminal care to a patient and his family. My previous skills of listening carefully to what is said and left unsaid during stressful, sad family situations came flooding back to me. It was such a relief to know I hadn't forgotten all my prior training.

PRACTICE ASSESSOR AND PRACTICE SUPERVISORS

Many of you will understand the support structure that exists in the clinical environment to meet the needs of students. In fact, you may have been mentors and will know the system which oversees and assesses students at different stages through their placement. Mentoring is a key process in facilitating learning. You all will likely remember the colleagues that supported you in your initial journeys up to and beyond registration. For each of us there are usually several key people who spring to mind as inspiring role models because they nurtured and guided us through.

It is recognised that the clinical placement provides students with vital opportunities to learn and develop. As registered nurses you have a responsibility under the NMC Code to actively pass on your knowledge and to teach students. Under the Standards to Support Learning and Assessment in Practice (SLAiP) (NMC 2008) mentors played multiple roles in facilitating learning, supervising and assessing students in the practice setting. It was a requirement that a student had supernumerary status and that 40% of their time was spent in working with their assigned mentor. Assessment was undertaken via direct observation, reflective discussion and writing and feedback from the wider team. There was a maintained register in each Trust which identified mentors and a more experienced 'sign-off mentor' who had met the additional NMC requirements of supervised scrutiny on three occasions to gain signing-off proficiency. The role of the sign-off mentor was to decide whether the student had achieved the required standards as a safe and competent practitioner.

However, these roles led to some problems as not all nurses were mentors, and workload allocation did not factor in the additional time needed to support this professional responsibility and process. Also, the ten-day preparation programme presented difficulties in some areas that were challenged with short staffing. The new Standards for Student Supervision and Assessment (SSSAs) (NMC 2018b) address these concerns in clear terms and focus on learning support, supervision and assessment of students both for pre-registration and Return to Practice. The standards cover three key areas:

- **Effective practice learning** reinforces that all students are supernumerary and all NMC registrants are actively involved in supporting students in their learning. It also highlights the importance of interprofessional learning and the involvement of patients and carers. Students are encouraged to be active participants in their learning journey.
- **Supervision of students** is now managed through a clear division of roles with the Practice Supervisor as teacher and the more senior Practice Assessor as the one who assesses and determines achievement. In conjunction with this the Academic Assessor will verify that learning outcomes have been met enabling the student to progress onwards.
- **Assessment of students and confirmation of proficiency** are the responsibilities of the approved educational institution and employing organisation. Effective, robust and objective evidence-based assessments must be in place. The support system provided by Practice Supervisor, Practice Assessor and Academic Assessor is key to helping students develop competence, confidence and be safe practitioners.

Whilst all NMC registrants have a responsibility to support you in practice, the Practice Supervisor will be your main link to the formative, or developmental, process of learning. In conjunction with the Supervisor, the Practice Assessor will make an objective assessment of your achievements in liaison with the Academic Assessor assigned by the university. It is proposed that this tripartite arrangement will facilitate effective learning in practice with supervision and assessment of proficiencies and competence acting as the cornerstones of process. Here are further details of the roles and responsibilities, with Figure 4.2 showing how the tripartite structure reinforces support and communication between staff and students:

Practice Supervisor

- Acts as a role model
- Supports learning whilst working within own scope of practice
- Possesses current knowledge and experience
- Contributes to assessment via feedback to Practice Assessor, recording experience of observing student in practice and raising any potential concerns

Practice Assessor

- Assesses achievement and provides feedback
- Works in partnership with the Academic Assessor and Practice Supervisors
- Gathers and co-ordinates feedback from the wider team
- Understands the student's learning needs and outcomes
- Possesses current knowledge and experience
- Undertakes preparation for the role, or provides evidence of prior experience that would facilitate the role

Academic Assessor

- Collates and confirms student achievement of programme outcomes in the academic environment
- Makes and records objective, evidence-based decisions on conduct, proficiency and achievement, and makes recommendations for progression
- Maintains current relevant knowledge and expertise
- Works in partnership with the nominated Practice Assessor
- Understands the student's learning and achievement in practice
- Communicates and collaborates with Academic and Practice Assessors at relevant points in the programme structure and student progression

(NMC SSSA 2018b)

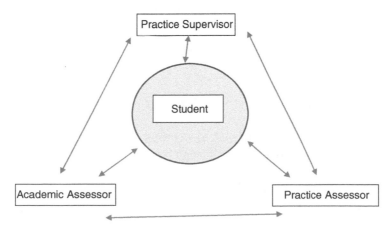

FIGURE 4.2   Tripartite support and assessment.

The Student–Supervisor–Assessor Relationship

> **Words of Wisdom**
>
> I found that developing a good working relationship and communicating effectively with both my assessor and supervisor aided my achievement of required outcomes. In hindsight I feel I was too hesitant to seek assistance and would recommend future students open lines of communication earlier and ask questions. I met with my assessor weekly to review my placement objectives. We built an easy rapport as we shared our thoughts on what had been achieved in the preceding days and what areas of work we should focus on next.

A determining factor in a successful return to the clinical setting lies in the relationship you cultivate with your Practice Assessor and Practice Supervisors. Try to establish rapport and understanding with placement staff from the outset as this will underpin and support the learning process. The clinical environment is busy and there will be many demands on your supervisor's time, so clear and effective communication on both sides is vital.

The full extent and nature of what you will need to accomplish may not be fully visible at the start, but an open and positive attitude will help to set the tone for good working relationships. Your allocated Supervisor or Assessor may not be in the clinical setting on your first day. They may be on leave, on a different shift or unwell: these things happen. Remember that you are joining a team and seek a friendly face who will take you under their wing. Learners thrive when they feel welcomed, and it does not always matter which specific staff member steps forward to take on this initial role (Scott and Spouse 2013). Indeed, settling in with the help of someone more junior can make for a gentler start.

Practical Arrangements

To achieve competence, you will need to demonstrate continuity. One of the first things to decide is how you plan to co-ordinate your time. To support and assess you, Practice Supervisors and Assessors will need to be with you so, for some of the time, you will need to arrange to be in the clinical placement when they are. There is a general understanding that students should commit to completing a minimum of two shifts or days each week. However, remember that students are supernumerary, and hours can be negotiated. Return to Practice programmes are inherently flexible to facilitate additional personal or family responsibilities. It is important to explain your individual situation, outlining any difficult days, planned holidays or other issues which you feel may have an impact. Whilst of course you will need to demonstrate professionalism and commitment, Assessors and Supervisors will work with you as much as they can.

Words of Wisdom

I decided that I would prefer to do just two days a week as I was concerned that it would take myself and my family some time to adjust. This allowed me time to do some other work for the course and work around my family life too. I also decided that if I did more placement hours at the beginning, I would have enough experiences for writing reflectively for the course essays.

Make every minute count. If your mentor has work responsibilities that you are unable to contribute to, ensure you have your placement handbook handy so you can be reviewing progress to date, make a list of your next queries, complete online educational modules or work through your reading list. I used placement time to complete online safeguarding and consent training whilst my mentor was otherwise engaged.

You will be completing between 150 and 450 supervised practice hours over a period of 4 to 6 months. Some courses may vary slightly. However, whatever the duration of your time in placement, it will go quickly. Good time management, therefore, is essential. Many returners counsel not to leave everything to the last minute. Try to pace yourself, setting goals for each day and week in practice so that you can mark progress and sustain momentum. Careful forward planning will help you to stay focused and enable a sense of partnership with your supervisors and assessor who will appreciate your initiative and organisation. Of course, there will always be days in the clinical setting when sudden events take over and plans go awry. These moments often call for quick and flexible thinking and this can be when Return to Practice students act instinctively, using their prior knowledge and skills to anticipate, respond and be supportive of others.

Learning Opportunities

Most returners will update their nursing skills in a single placement which offers a range of learning opportunities. Some of these will take the student beyond the physical confines of the core practice setting. You may find yourself spending time with specialist nurses and other healthcare professionals including physiotherapists, occupational therapists, nursery nurses and social workers. A day spent with a community team will complement an inpatient acute placement; time in theatres will help to make sense of the patient's journey through surgery; attending carers' meetings will inform you about partnership working; a morning with the ward clerk or receptionist will provide insight into the administrative processes around care and treatment, and so on.

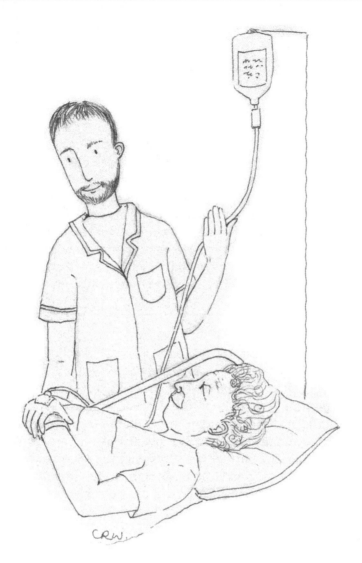

ILLUSTRATION NO. 4.1B   Gaining confidence.

Words of Wisdom

I worked out that assessors and supervisors are there to assist you with your learn-ing and assess your competence in practice. They are not necessarily going to direct your learning or provide learning opportunities for you – you may need to do this yourself. Be proactive in getting involved in as many things as possible, attending MDT meetings, asking to tag along with physios and OTs, volunteering to observe or take part in procedures – in essence, make the most of the opportunity.

I was attached to a community matron for my placement. We used travelling time in the car between patients to discuss the nursing care given and to answer my numerous questions.

CONFIDENCE AND COMPETENCE

Your first few weeks in placement are a time for settling in and acclimatising. We have seen from Maslow's hierarchy of needs that an environment needs to feel friendly and supportive before it can become conducive to learning (Maslow and Lewis 1987). Many returners find a comfort zone for their first few days – a place of safety where they feel in control. This could be a physical place such as a hospital sluice, an activity such as providing personal care or a role such as shadowing and observing a member of staff. These are starting positions giving you time to get to know people and take stock of your new surroundings. It is from this steady state that confidence levels can start to grow. What is vital here is to recognise that at some point you do need to move on. Comfort zones offer very limited challenges and if we stay in them too long, we can become stagnant and resistant to change. To progress, and achieve self-efficacy, we need to step beyond to a zone of slight discomfort where there are demands and risks, but also the potential for development and achievement (White 2008). White calls this 'the optimal performance zone' and presents a dynamic of constant movement so that change and risk is always there but at manageable levels. He cautions that if we move too quickly, however, we can find ourselves in a danger zone where the stresses feel too great and can threaten to overwhelm us. Figure 4.3 represents his model. He links his ideas to the way in which teams adapt and change which we explored earlier in this chapter (Tuckman 1965).

Returning to student status can be both liberating and isolating. Hughes-Morris and Roberts (2017) state that when qualified practitioners return to being students, they can feel scrutinised and vulnerable. Although their study focused on mature nurses embarking on Specialist Community Public Health (SCPHN) training, their findings have some relevance to the experience of nurses re-entering their profession. There is a shared sense of self-questioning and a self-consciousness about how to behave back in the student role. What is also clear for both student groups is that when practice teams recognise and acknowledge pre-existing skills and knowledge, nurse returners and SCPHN students can start to feel their confidence and

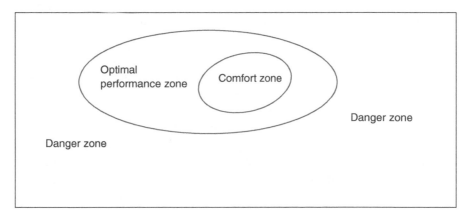

FIGURE 4.3 Comfort Zone Model. *Source:* Adapted from White 2008.

competence grow (Hughes-Morris and Roberts 2017; Coates and Macfadyen 2021). Many enjoy the challenge of being a student again, relishing the opportunity to learn new things and rediscover parts of themselves which they may not have used for a while. Eraut's key research (2007) into workplace learning is relevant here: he discusses how confidence can only grow when sufficient challenge (but not too much) is in equal balance with supportive feedback. This is a recurrent concept in mentoring and echoes earlier key work by Daloz (1986) who argued that professional growth requires both nurturing and challenging. Those of you who have mentored before in your previous nursing life, or who may have supported people in other types of workplaces, will understand this dynamic.

Words of Wisdom

Becoming a student again and being constantly supervised is challenging.
Being a student in placement and feeling scrutinised can be intense and unsettling.
Getting people to understand what the course involves is key.
Mentors don't always have enough time for you, and some do seem challenged by RTP students.
Enjoy your placement and the challenge of new learning!
It is important to understanding your limitations as RTP student in terms of scope of practice.
I did become frustrated towards end of placement because I was unable to complete all areas of care independently whilst still a student.
My brain felt reawakened!
It is important to take constructive criticism positively.

Knowing when and how to motivate a student to take on more responsibility is an important skill as is being able to give constructive criticism. We have touched on the importance of self-awareness, and in the next chapter we will look at the Johari Window, an invaluable tool to help keep this aspect of personal development alive and in continuous growth. One of its key messages concerns the art of receiving constructive feedback. Through listening and understanding sometimes difficult to receive responses from those around us – be they friends or assessors! – we see ourselves through the eyes of others. It can be an uncomfortable experience, but once our emotions settle, new insights often emerge. We learn more about ourselves and our impact on others from this kind of honest, balanced feedback.

In practice placements, you will receive responses from many quarters, including patients, carers and members of the multi-disciplinary team. All are invaluable in providing a range of perspectives and helping you to gauge your own practice development. Regular informal feedback from supervisors and assessors may be delivered verbally on a day-by-day basis. Try to ask for this commentary, cultivating a proactive approach to your own learning. Initiating a request for feedback can be empowering for both student and mentor, enhancing a trusting relationship and establishing good practice for re-entry to the nursing workforce (Allen and Molloy 2017). Midpoints mark a significant time for more formal written review where achievement can be recognised, and attention re-directed to any remaining objectives. Active listening is an essential skill for the giver and receiver of constructive feedback, ensuring that both are fully engaged in the process (Hardavella et al. 2017).

Words of Wisdom

Initially the placement went well; I was enjoying being back in a nursing environment, but I began to feel like I was shadowing staff but not getting anywhere. I needed to take ownership of the situation and ask myself why. After discussion with my assessor, I asked to take on my own caseload of patients, under supervision. This turned out to be just what I needed. My confidence grew from then and the learning opportunities came to me naturally. I was very lucky to have a practice assessor that knew when to give me a push to do more and encouraged me to take on more each shift.

A skilled supervisor or assessor will know how to encourage and motivate, sensing when students need to challenge themselves further. However, as we know from our own nursing experiences, mentors are busy people who will have competing priorities and sometimes very little time. As a student, therefore, it is crucial to cultivate a positive mindset and a resourceful approach. This is probably impossible on your first day when you may well feel swamped or buffeted, and certainly not in control. Let your first week be what it will be but resolve to try to grasp things firmly once you have a sense of what is happening around you.

Words of Wisdom

Don't be afraid to ask questions – there is so much support for you at every level.
Be positive. Challenge yourself.
Grasp the clinical experience with both hands and ask the thick questions!
Be assertive – take all opportunities offered.
Believe in yourself and be assertive.
Ask; don't wait to be asked. Be prepared to speak up.
Be bold; don't be scared – have self-belief; remember what a great job nursing is.
Be proactive with your mentors because they are very busy.
Be confident about getting signed off.
Fully commit to doing whatever it takes to complete the course.
Be prepared for hard work.
Make the most of the opportunity.

It is vital to ask questions. As we have already discussed, every returner comes with a unique background and a different set of skills. Some pre-registration students may also be mature learners, and some will have past or current jobs in healthcare settings but, because they are not qualified nurses, they offer their mentors a 'blank canvas' with respect to practice learning. This is not true for returners: their task is to support their mentors to understand what they need to learn, and this can only be done effectively through questioning and discussion. This is an active process which will help both student and supervisor to bring into focus objectives and priorities. It will require you to be assertive at times, and this is not easy in student mode. It helps to remember that every question, however simplistic, will contribute to a clearer picture of your learning needs and serve to foster relationships. Often returners and mentors come to enjoy a sharing of skills and a reciprocity that rewards each with a sense of personal growth (Grossman 2012). By the end of your placement, you will feel more like a colleague, working alongside others, contributing to the interactions necessary for effective clinical reasoning and responding to their needs for supportive feedback (Higgs et al. 2019; Coates and Macfadyen 2021).

Words of Wisdom from a Practice Assessor

Supporting a Return to Practice student gave me the opportunity to revisit areas of practice that I had not thought about for some time. It also made me reflect on areas of my own practice that I could do some revision around. It also made me think about the levels of support that are needed for different students. Return to practice is mostly about confidence building and reassurance as the student has a wealth of experience and knowledge which just needs reawakening.

DECISION MAKING AND LEADERSHIP

Many returners describe a key moment in their practice placement when things click back into place. It may be that they are able to respond quickly and effectively to an unexpected practice situation such as calming an angry relative or caring for a patient who has suffered a fall. Sometimes the moment comes when another member of staff seeks you out for advice. As you progress through your placement, supervision becomes more 'long arm' enabling you to demonstrate the ability to lead and make autonomous clinical decisions.

We will expand on these important higher-level proficiencies by way of two examples from recent returners. In both accounts we see them showing initiative, working collaboratively, and taking responsibility for their own decision making. The first extract shows how a child nurse returner used her clinical judgement when caring for an eighteen-month-old child with bronchiolitis. The patient was receiving oxygen therapy via nasal prongs. Vital signs were being monitored every hour using a Paediatric Early Warning Score (PEWS). This assessment tool is used to record observations and standardise decision-making responses (Royal College of Paediatrics & Child Health 2019). We can see that she follows logical steps, processing information and deducing the best course of action based on her observations and the PEWS score. She also senses that her intuition has a part to play.

Returner's Account

On examination I noted that whilst most of his vital signs were within range for his age and scoring a zero on the PEWS chart, his respiratory rate was triggering a 1 and was noticeably faster than I would expect for a child of his age. Normal respiratory pattern is an easy, relaxed, subconscious activity at a rate dependent on the age and activity of the child (Hazinski 2013). I had counted 48 breaths per minute with a notable increased work of breathing with some intercostal recession visible. For his age and guided by the PEWS tool, a respiratory rate of 20–35 breaths per minute would have been within expected range. Assessing a child and identifying any change in condition is fundamental to the nursing role. Respiratory rates have been identified as one of the most important clinical signs observed in children, as it can direct care to alleviate life-threatening symptoms. Children's conditions can change drastically quickly so I understood the importance of responding promptly to the findings of my assessment (Jones et al. 2014). I was concerned that this child was deteriorating, and my gut instinct told me to inform not just my supervisor but also the nurse in charge and the paediatric registrar who was on the ward at the time. I felt this child would need some intervention and further support. My clinical judgement came from analytical reasoning; however, it is possible that I also made the decision to escalate his care intuitively based on my past experience and knowledge. A recent study concluded that intuition in clinical practice should be used to support decision making as this increases quality and safety of patient care (Melin-Johansson et al. 2017). These strategies are not mutually exclusive: both involve pattern or cue recognition (Benner 2001).

When we think of leadership, senior roles come to mind. Some of you will be returning to practice having worked before as nurse managers or team leaders. However, a view of nursing today requires us all to develop leadership skills. Leadership and management are not the same thing. Basset, chair of the RCN nurses in management and leadership forum, explains that 'managing is about delivering, while leadership is about direction' (Bassett in Evans 2022, p. 18).

Management focuses attention on the use of skills to plan or organise resources, whereas leadership is about engaging with others and fostering change. Spector (2014) proposes that a common theme that reoccurs when defining leadership is that of influencing the attitudes, beliefs and behaviours of others. Nurses are needed as role models for future healthcare practice, our behaviours and skills setting an example for evidence-based, person-centred care. These qualities are eloquently illustrated by one returning student who reflected on her experience of supporting a healthcare assistant. Although new to the clinical setting and only just starting to recover her own confidence and competence, she demonstrates excellent leadership skills in helping the staff member to feel needed and valued.

Returner's Account

'One of the main functions of a leader is the development of others' (Ellis 2019). This account will focus on this area of leadership, demonstrating my competence in delegation and encouraging the professional development of a Health Care Assistant (HCA) working within my team. The HCA was an agency employee whom I had not met before. She asked me if she could do anything to help with patient care. I asked if she was qualified to undertake patient observations, and she informed me that she had been trained but had not had much experience and did not feel confident. We therefore agreed to work collaboratively carrying out the observations so I could assess her skills and developmental needs. After the assessment, support was given by demonstrating how best to take a patient's respiration rate and how to accurately record the results on the National Early Warning Score (NEWS) 2 chart (Royal College of Physicians 2017). After competently carrying out the observations under supervision, she reported feeling confident to practise the skills by herself. I ascertained that she knew the importance of reporting any abnormal findings to me straight away as research clearly indicates that abnormal vital signs are associated with poor patient outcome and intervening before harm occurs is central to the role of the nurse (Johnson et al. 2017). We then followed up with an evaluation on progress. The observations had been carried out correctly and she told me that she felt much more confident and empowered as a result.

When leading individuals, a flexible approach is needed to make the most of the contribution of others involved in providing patient care. Patient safety must always be the primary focus. I have learnt that collective leadership means everyone has leadership responsibility and it is not exclusive to more formal positions in healthcare. Registered nurses provide leadership by acting as a role model for best practice in the delivery of nursing care (NMC 2018). By inspiring others to do the best they can by doing the best you can yourself, we can create compassionate, nurturing cultures for the health and well-being of patients, colleagues, and ourselves.

Also apparent in this account are those soft skills we discussed earlier. A contemporary view of leadership is one of compassion embracing often unseen qualities such as listening, enabling and empathy (Quinn 2017). It involves seeking feedback and sharing learning with others. Feather (2009) states that effective leadership rests on emotional intelligence, pointing out that recognising and expressing our own emotions helps us to connect with the feelings of those around us.

As one of the most versatile healthcare professions, nursing encompasses many transferable skills. Honed over the course of careers, we perhaps have come to overlook the importance of being able to manage time, problem solve and help others to make sense of experiences. Without doubt, we all use these skills in our everyday family lives, whether that be strategies for peace keeping or negotiation! A degree of self-awareness will show us that these same skills transfer back into the workplace, opening up job opportunities and progression into specialities.

However, at the start of your journey back into the profession you may welcome some updating in these areas. A wide range of courses, workshops and resources are available via the Florence Nightingale Academy, the NHS Leadership Academy, the Royal College of Nursing, NHS England and Health Education England regions. We have included their websites in our reference list at the end of the chapter. Framed within the premise that anyone who finds a better way of doing things is being a leader, the NHS Leadership Academy was established to support healthcare staff to discover and develop their potential. The programmes offer flexibility and progression through stages of personal leadership development from initial foundations through to senior levels (NHS Leadership Academy 2018). Nurses are seen as change agents for healthcare provision, and therefore need to be supported to develop the skills required to undertake this responsibility.

Return to Practice courses provide opportunities for discussion if you are keen to resume or pursue a more senior role once re-registered. Some Trusts provide their own training, or they may offer support and funding for leadership development. Annual work appraisals and reflective discussions during the NMC re-validation process are also occasions to discuss continuous professional development.

UNDERSTANDING SCOPE OF PRACTICE AND YOUR CHOSEN FIELD

In Chapter 2 we outlined the NMC Future Nurse Standards of proficiency for registered nurses (2018). They are of course at the core of your placement experience and so here we have unpacked them further. We encourage you to read them in full on the NMC website which we have referenced at the end of this chapter.

Platforms and annexes	Registered nurses in all fields must be...
Platform 1 **Being an accountable professional**	...responsible for providing care that is person-centred and evidence based. This platform links to the personal and professional values stipulated in the NMC Code including compassion, accountability, communication and the prioritising of those in our care. We must also act as reflective practitioners.
Platform 2 **Promoting health and preventing ill health**	...involved in improving and maintaining the mental, physical and behavioural health of people. Nurses must be able to advise and support individuals from all age groups and in all care settings to make healthy choices to maximise their quality of life. They must possess skills and knowledge in teaching and health promotion.

(continued)

(continued)

Platforms and annexes	Registered nurses in all fields must be...
Platform 3 **Assessing needs and planning care**	*...able to prioritise the holistic needs of people, ensuring care provided is evidence-based and person-centred.*
Platform 4 **Providing and evaluating care**	*...able to work in partnership with people across all age ranges and settings, ensuring care is safe, effective and of a high standard and that desired outcomes are met.*
Platform 5 **Leading and managing nursing care and working in teams**	*...responsible for managing and leading nursing care, delegating appropriately and communicating effectively across a diverse range of situations. They must be active, equal and collaborative members of the interdisciplinary team.*
Platform 6 **Improving safety and quality of care**	*...actively involved in risk assessment and quality improvement. They must prioritise the best interests and needs of those in their care.*
Platform 7 **Coordinating care**	*...aware of local and national policies, playing a leadership role in managing and integrating people's care needs across their life span. They must have an understanding of organisational change management.*
Annexe A **Communication and relationship management skills**	*...be able to demonstrate the ability to communicate compassionately and manage safely relationships with people of all ages, including families and carers.*
Annexe B **Nursing procedures**	*...be able to demonstrate achievement of identified proficiencies. It is acknowledged that the level of expertise will vary according to nurse's chosen field of practice.*

At present, most RTP SCPHN courses have been approved to run in compliance with the 2004 SCPHN standards (NMC 2004). However, the NMC have recently published new standards so this situation will change as courses realign (NMC 2022). If you are a SCPHN practitioner planning to return to practice over the next few years, we would advise that you consult the NMC website and talk to course providers so that you are able to understand what might be involved.

We also discussed in Chapter 2 how the NMC Future Nurse standards (2018) herald a vision of the contemporary nurse with a broader and deeper scope of practice, equipped to care for people of all ages and backgrounds. Pre-registration nurse curricula address these requirements with students undertaking more advanced clinical skills training such as venepuncture and engaging in topics relevant to all four nursing fields.

For nurse returners this change poses challenges. Most have years of experience in their field of nursing, and many are highly specialised practitioners within that area. However, the NMC require those returning to the profession to achieve the benchmark set by these revised nursing proficiencies. This means that the journey to join the current workforce involves not just retrieving existing skills but also learning new ones. This is not necessarily negative nor impossible, but it does place greater demand both on student and course provider. In the next section we will see that the practice assessment document used for return to practice is aligned and reflects the generic nature of the Future Nurse standards (as required by the NMC 2018). The practice placement, on the other hand, remains field specific to match the returning nurse's prior experience. Key phrases – 'intended area of practice' and 'intended scope of practice' – within the NMC Standards for Return to Practice programmes (2019) acknowledge this fine balance and offer some clarity. Scope of practice is an important term and key tenet for all healthcare professionals because it defines individual safe and effective practice (Health & Care Professions Council 2021; NMC 2018a). Our NMC Code (NMC 2018a) states that we must work only within the limits of our competence and knowledge, raising immediate concerns if asked to extend beyond our nursing role or training. Notwithstanding the fixed outer boundaries of supervised practice and student status, it can be difficult for returners to know their scope of practice because it will be constantly on the move as prior skills and knowledge are remembered and begin to fuse with new learning. However, it is recognised that achievement of practice proficiencies will play out on different levels according to an individual returner's field of nursing and prior experience. Provision is made for students to address some areas of proficiency through hypothetical discussion or simulation.

A key conclusion from the Francis Report (Francis 2013) and highlighted by Smith (2012) is that for patients to feel safe and cared for, the healthcare professional carrying out the work must feel safe and cared for too. As individuals we have a responsibility to be mindful of our own vulnerability which could impact on our performance and increase the risk of errors. Scope of practice is about our safety too. Reason's three-bucket model (Figure 4.4) helps us to identify if we are in danger of compromising our patients or ourselves (Reason 2004). This tool is memorable, and simple to use and share, enabling team members to support each other and work

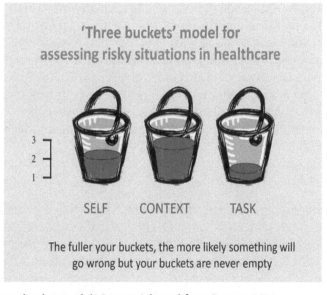

'Three buckets' model for assessing risky situations in healthcare

3
2
1

SELF   CONTEXT   TASK

The fuller your buckets, the more likely something will go wrong but your buckets are never empty

FIGURE 4.4 Three-bucket model. *Source:* Adapted from Reason 2004.

more effectively. The first bucket contains everything related to **self** and asks us to assess factors such as tiredness, stress, hunger, running late for work, feeling preoccupied or unwell. The second bucket relates to **context** – the situation we are in – with questions such as: Is the area understaffed or under resourced? Is there a lack of leadership? Are the expectations unrealistic? Finally, the **task** bucket gauges the difficulty or unfamiliarity of the specific activity facing you. The greater the level in each bucket the higher the risk of errors occurring. The concept of buckets is much in use when it comes to measuring stress; we will return to another one in a later chapter!

HOW WILL I BE ASSESSED?

Any kind of exam or test tends to strike fear and anxiety in us all. However, most assessments form part of a process, and returning to practice is no exception. Assessments can be formative and summative. You may recall that formative means developmental – a kind of practice run designed to test out something in a safe way that invites helpful feedback and informs later attempts. Summative is the final assessment which fixes achievement as a pass or fail.

The first step is self-assessment which usually starts during course inductions. As we have discussed previously, this has always been recognised as important in helping returners to gauge their gap in practice, thereby setting the pace and focus for learning in the clinical setting. Self-assessment, evaluation or appraisal is now a requirement within the nursing workforce. We provided an example of a self-assessment and development tool in Chapter 3, the kind of which are now being adopted by universities to formalise this activity in line with NMC Future Nurse standards (2018).

Practice Assessors and Supervisors will look to you for guidance in terms of what you are hoping to achieve in the early days. Your self-assessment will be a crucial part of the overall placement assessment because it helps everyone to identify and focus on your key learning needs, highlighting areas of strength and pointing to what will need more support. In your first meeting with your Practice Assessor, you will be able to arrange learning opportunities and plan how best to pace your practice assessments. Remember that you are likely to spend more of your time with Practice Supervisors who will liaise with your Practice Assessor, reporting on your progress. It is important to note, however, that you may not be shadowing or working with supervisors throughout entire shifts as they may well have other responsibilities to fulfil too.

Words of Wisdom

I found that identifying and meeting my assessor and supervisor individually at the start to discuss previous experience and sort out working together was really beneficial. Then I arranged to meet them again soon after to go through the requirements of the practice assessment as in the beginning I found it all too overwhelming and a bit off putting!

Be familiar with placement objectives and share proactive responsibility for achieving them with your supervisor or assessor. Agree the frequency, dates and times of both the informal and formally stipulated review meetings at the placement start. If a meeting is missed, for whatever reason, make plans as soon as possible for when it can be rescheduled. Assume weekly responsibility for personally reviewing your objectives. Write short prompt notes outlining the evidence to demonstrate which objectives you believe have been achieved to date to inform your review meeting discussions.

Be aware of your assessor's planned clinical work for the following week. Where can you maximise learning opportunities to meet outstanding objectives? Consider background reading you can suggest or undertake to meet objectives that may be hard to attain in your placement. Be flexible in your approach – if there are gaps in your learning experience, could shadowing a fellow professional be arranged if appropriate?

Remember supervisors and assessors are busy people. Therefore, help make their job easier by arriving at review sessions well prepared, focused and enthusiastic whilst proactively assuming joint responsibility to make the placement a success.

Practice Assessment Documentation

Assessments are recorded in a Practice Assessment Document (PAD). The proficiency outcomes contained within this document identify the knowledge, skills, attitudes and behaviours that a returning nurse must demonstrate by the end of the course. They are organised with reference to the relevant NMC standards of proficiency (NMC 2018; NMC 2004). PADs will differ in layout and structure from course to course, but all include the essential elements required and approved by the NMC, with most Return to Nursing PADs aligning closely with the platforms and annexes found in the Future Nurse standards (NMC 2018). Here we have outlined a typical example of the assessment elements based on the England Practice Assessment Document for Return to Practice Nursing Programme (by *kind permission from* the PAN England Return to Practice Learning Group 2020).

Summative elements of practice assessment	What you are required to demonstrate
Professional Values Based on the NMC Code (MNC 2018)	All areas of your practice are underpinned and comply with identified professional values.
Practice Proficiencies Based on the seven platforms and two annexes (NMC 2018)	You have achieved required proficiencies. *Achievement of some may take place through hypothetical discussions or simulation.*
Medicines Management Based on Annexe B: Nursing procedures	A single summative assessment of your knowledge and competence in safely administering medication for a group of patients within the practice environment. *It must be preceded by formative assessments or 'practice runs'.*

(continued)

(continued)

Summative elements of practice assessment	What you are required to demonstrate
Episode of Care 1 Holistic assessment based on progression across several platforms.	A single summative assessment of your supervision and teaching of a junior learner (student, carer or service user) in practice, based on the delivery of direct person-centred care. It must be preceded by formative assessments or 'practice runs'.
Episode of Care 2 Holistic assessment based on the seven platforms.	A single summative assessment of your organisation and management of care for a group or caseload of people with complex care covering all seven platforms. It must be preceded by formative assessments or 'practice runs'.

Assessment of your proficiency is undertaken by a combination of direct observation of your practice, discussion about your involvement in care activities and feedback from the wider team, service users and carers. As we have already highlighted, mid-points mark a crucial juncture because they provide the opportunity for formative feedback and an acknowledgement of progress. There will also be a review of your assessment documentation and discussion about your self-reflections on practice. At the end of your placement there will be a summative assessment in terms of your proficiencies to ensure that you are a safe competent practitioner. This may seem daunting; however, the manner of assessment follows a traditional format which has not changed very much over the years. The terminology and paperwork are different, but our responsibility and accountability to patients remain a constant. We are duty bound to deliver safe and effective care. This is a journey, and you will have time, opportunity and support to regain your confidence and achieve success in meeting all the required outcomes. Whilst there may be small variations in Return to Practice courses nationwide, basic placement processes are likely to be similar and are outlined here.

Placement process	
Prior to placement	Returner contacts placement. Practice Assessor and Supervisors allocated.
Introductory and orientation	Self-assessment discussed and learning opportunities planned. Review of proficiencies and orientation checklist completed.
Initial meeting	Learning and development needs identified and planned.
Midpoint meeting	Review of progress and acknowledgement of achievement so far. Remaining future learning and development needs identified.
Final meeting	Progress and achievement recorded. Final assessment and decision.

95.8% of students successfully complete their return to nursing, and 100% of these nurses go on to secure employment (Health Education England 2014). However, it must be recognised that things do not always go as planned. Two attempts are offered for summative assessments. If a student is unable to demonstrate required levels of competency the first time around, a second opportunity is offered providing an alternative practice placement can be arranged. Of course, it is disappointing to fail; however, there is no shame in needing another opportunity. Often it is a matter of being able to convey a sense of confidence in practice and for some this can just take a little longer to achieve.

Course failure does occur, but again this happens to very few and is usually anticipated. Non-attendance in placement or concerns about safe practice can signal a poor outcome. Even then, however, efforts will always be made to help students to turn things around. Very infrequently, a student may feel that nursing is no longer the right destination. Return to Practice courses are a test run. It may be that too many changes have taken place in healthcare settings, or the stresses of the nursing role have rendered the experience one of discomfort or even foreboding. It must be said that the number of returners who leave in this way is very small. A slightly larger percentage may step away because of mistiming their return, perhaps because of too many other competing commitments.

Sometimes the journey back to nursing can take longer than expected. Difficult family circumstances or personal ill health can trigger the need for time out. This can be accommodated by universities in the form of extensions, mitigating circumstances processes or study breaks. Most courses have inbuilt flexibility to support students in this situation. On rare occasions some may decide on a course withdrawal; however, it is heartening and not uncommon for us to see such individuals re-apply at a future time when life feels more manageable.

YOUR SUPPORT NETWORKS

Returning to practice is a brave step and your friends and families will want to rally round to help. It can be hard to accept support especially when you are used to being in the assisting role. However, now is the time to ask for what you need, remembering perhaps that this may give others a chance to repay your past kindnesses. There will be course pinch points when academic assignments collide with practice assessments: forward planning so that you have extra support through these busy times can make all the difference.

We have spoken often about the invaluable part played by peer support. Every cohort of returners seems to bond quickly, and some people go on to foster lasting friendships. This camaraderie strengthens when students start their practice placement. Whilst formal support networks within organisations play a vital role, empathy and reassurance may come most usefully from those who are sharing this journey with you. Nowadays, supportive contact is likely to come via instant messaging services as well as face-to-face during study days.

Words of Wisdom

Give each other support and don't give up.

Make the most of peer support and do not worry if others seem ahead.

Remember your scope of practice – be strong enough to say when you can't do things.

Don't worry about the course! It can build up to seem massive, but best to take your time and go with it.

Don't be afraid to ask for help.

Learn from feedback and use all the resources around you.

Try not to be too self-critical.

You will get through it; you will meet lots of lovely people with the same worries and fears as you.

Exchange phone numbers with others on the course so that you can keep each other going.

Set yourself small goals each day and tick them off as you go along!

Don't give up when you feel it is too much – hang in there! – it is achievable.

We have endeavoured to map out the route back to clinical practice, sketching in some contours and features we feel you are likely to encounter. However, the truth is that every returning journey is unique. This is both a professional and personal transition, coloured and shaped by who you are, your past nursing roles and achievements, your life experiences, and your future goals. The level of challenge and ease can vary from week to week and from placement to placement. Making sense of these twists and turns is important and a good way to do this is in writing. These early notes may be lists, jottings or odds and ends, but they will help you to mark significant days, de-brief times of difficulty and signal future learning. Some students have found it useful to keep a diary of their thoughts and feelings, making a log of experiences as they go through their placement. Others keep brief records of each day, key words which will jog their memory when they come to discuss achievements with their Practice Assessor. The last word goes to one returner who neatly sums up this advice.

Words of Wisdom

Tip – Take a pocket notebook everywhere with you, to jot things down you can later look up and to note down events and experiences in practice to get used to reflection and critical thinking. Even if the event seems small, it can be surprising how many different dimensions of reflection and learning can come from it!

REFERENCES

Allen, L. and Molloy, E. (2017). The influence of a preceptor-student 'Daily Feedback Tool' on clinical feedback practices in nursing education: a qualitative study. *Nurse Education Today* 49: 57–62.

Belbin Associates (2006). Belbin team roles (online). Available at: www.belbin.com.

Belbin, M. (1981). *Management in Teams*, 3e. Oxford: Elsevier Limited.

Benner, P. (2001). *From Novice to Expert. Excellence and Power in Clinical Nursing Practice*, Commemorative Edition. New Jersey: Prentice Hall Health.

Benner, P. (2005). Using the Dreyfus model of skill acquisition to describe and interpret skill acquisition and clinical judgment in nursing practice and education. *The Bulletin of Science, Technology and Society Special Issue: Human Expertise in the Age of the Computer* 24 (3): 188–199.

Benner, P. (2010). *Preface To: Transitions Theory: Middle Range and Situation Specific Theories in Nursing Research and Practice*. New York: Springer Publishing Company.

Coates, M. and Macfadyen, A. (2021). Student experiences of a return to practice programme: a qualitative study. *British Journal of Nursing* 30 (15): 900–908.

Daloz, L.A. (1986). *Effective Teaching and Mentorship: Realizing the Transformational Power of Adult Learning Expefriences*, 209–235. San Francisco: Jossey-Bass.

Ellis, P. (2019). *Leadership, Management and Teamworking in Nursing, 3e*. Learning Matters: Sage.

Eraut, M. (2007). Learning from other people in the workplace. *Oxford Review of Education* 33 (4): 403–422.

Evans, N. (2022). How you can develop your leadership skills. *Nursing Management* 29 (2): 14–15.

Feather, R. (2009). Emotional intelligence in relation to nursing leadership: does it matter? *Journal of Nursing Management* 17: 376–382.

Francis, R. (2013). The Mid Staffordshire NHS Foundation Trust Public Inquiry. Available at: http://www.midstaffspublicinquiry.com.

Goleman, D. (2020). *Emotional Intelligence. Why It Can Matter More than IQ*. London: Bloomsbury Publishing PLC.

Grossman, S. (2012). *Mentoring in Nursing. A Dynamic and Collaborative Process*. New York: Springer Publishing Company LLC.

Hardavella, G., Aamli-Gaagnat, A., Saad, N. et al. (2017). How to give and receive feedback effectively. *Breathe* 13: 327–333.

Hazinski (2013). *Normal respiratory rates in children*. https://media.gosh.nhs.uk/documents/Normal_Respiratory_Rates_in_Children.pdf.

Health and Care Professions Council (HCPC) (2021). https://www.hcpc-uk.org/standards/meeting-our-standards/scope-of-practice

Health Education England (2014). Nursing return to practice: review of the current landscape.

Higgs, J., Jensen, G.M., Loftus, S., and Christensen, N. (2019). *Clinical Reasoning in the Health Professions.* Elsevier Ltd.

Hughes, A.M., Gregory, M.E., Joseph, D.L. et al. (2016). Saving lives: a meta-analysis of team training in healthcare. *Journal of Applied Psychology* 101 (9): 1266.

Hughes-Morris, D. and Roberts, D. (2017). transition to SCPHN; the effects of returning to student status on autonomous practitioners. *British Journal of School Nursing* 12 (5): 234–243.

Johnson,K. D., Mueller, L., and Winkelman, C. (2017). The nurse response to abnormal vital sign recording in the emergency department. *Journal of Clinical Nursing* 26 (1–2): 148–156.

Jones, C.H.D., Neill, S., Lakhanpaul,M., Roland, D., Singlehurst-Mooney, H., and Thompson, M. (2014). Information needs of parents for acute childhood illness: determining 'what, how, where and when' of safety netting using a qualitative exploration with parents and clinicians. *BMJ Open.* https://bmjopen.bmj.com/content/bmjopen/4/1/e003874.full.pdf

Lewin, K. (1947). Group decision and social change. *Readings in Social Psychology* 3 (1): 197–211.

Maslow, A. and Lewis, K.J. (1987). Maslow's hierarchy of needs. *Salenger Incorporated* 14 (17): 987–990.

Meleis, A.I. (2010). *Transitions Theory: Middle Range and Situation Specific Theories in Nursing Research and Practice.* New York: Springer Publishing Company.

Melin-Johansson, C., Palmqvist, R., and Ronnberg, L. (2017). Clinical intuition in the nursing process and decision-making – A mixed-studies review. *Journal of Clinical Nursing* 26 (23–24):3936–3949.

Morton-Cooper, A. (1989). *Returning to Nursing. A Guide for Nurses and Health Visitors.* London: Macmillan Education Ltd.

Myers, S. (2013). Team Dynamics-how they affect performance.

NMC (2018). Future Nurse. Standards of proficiency for registered Nurses. NMC.

NHS Leadership Academy (2018). Available at: https://www.leadershipacademy.nhs.uk.

NMC (2004). *Standards of Proficiency for Pre-Registration Nursing Education.* London: NMC.

NMC (2008). *Standards to Support Learning and Assessment in Practice (Slaip).* London: NMC.

NMC (2018a). *The Code. Professional Standards of Practice and Behaviour for Nurses, Midwives and Nursing Associates.* NMC.

NMC (2018b). *Part 2 Standards for Student Supervision and Assessment (SSSA).* NMC.

NMC (2022). Standards of proficiency for specialist community public health nurses. NMC.

PAN England Return to Practice Learning Group (2020). England practice assessment document for return to practice nursing programme.

Quinn, B. (2017). Role of nursing leadership in providing compassionate care. *Nursing Standard* 32 (16–19).

Reason, J. (2004). Beyond the organisational accident: the need for 'error wisdom' on the frontline. *Quality & Safety in Health Care* 13 (Suppl. 2): ii28–i33.

Robinson, O.J., Vytal, K., Cornwell, B.R., and Grillon, C. (2013). The impact of anxiety upon cognition: perspectives from human threat of shock studies. *Frontiers in Human Neuroscience* 7: 203.

Royal College of Physicians (2017). National Early Warning Score (NEWS) 2: standardising the assessment of acute-illness severity in the NHS.

Royal College of Paediatrics and Child Health (2019). *Paediatric Early Warning System (PEW System) – Developing a Standardised Tool in England*. RCPCH.

Scott, I. and Spouse, J. (2013). *Practice-Based Learning in Nursing, Health and Social Care: Mentorship, Facilitation and Supervision*. Wiley Blackwell.

Smith, P. (2012). *The Emotional Labour of Nursing Revisited: Can Nurses Still Care?* Bloomsbury Publishing.

Spector, B. (2014). Flawed from the 'get-go': lee Iacocca and the origins of transformational leadership. *Leadership* 10 (3): 361–379.

Stevens, J. (2014). Support for nurses returning to practice. *Nursing Times* 110 (48): 12–14.

Thistlethwaite, J.E. (2012). *Values-based Interprofessional Collaborative Practice: Working Together in Health Care*. Cambridge University Press.

Tuckman, B.W. (1965). Development sequence in small groups. *Psychological Bulletin* 63 (6): 384–399. 1965.

West, M., Armit, K., Lowenthal, L. et al. (2015). *Leadership and Leadership Development in Health Care: The Evidence Base*. The Kings Fund.

White, A. (2008). *From Comfort Zone to Performance Management. Understanding Development and Performance*. Belgium: White and Maclean Publishing.

USEFUL WEBSITES

The Florence Nightingale Academy. Website: https://theflorence.academy.

NHS Leadership Academy (2018). https://www.leadershipacademy.nhs.uk.

NHS England. Website: https://www.england.nhs.uk.

The Royal College of Nursing. website: https://www.rcn.org.uk.

CHAPTER 5

Reflective Practice

STORIES

'My first practice placement was on a medical ward in a busy teaching hospital. I had had no previous experience of healthcare so was feeling very new to everything. We were looking after a lady who I will call May (not her real name). May was elderly with diabetes and heart problems. She had just had a bath and was making her way back to her bed area with the help of two physiotherapy assistants. Suddenly she collapsed on to the floor! I did not know what had happened. I was aware that people were rushing towards her and that she was not moving. Curtains were drawn around bed areas and the crash team came running on to the ward with equipment. I was asked to look after the other patients, so I went to sit with an elderly lady in the bay who looked frightened. A little later between the gaps in the curtains I could see May lying on her bed. She was still wearing her pink fluffy slippers – the same ones which I had helped her to put on that morning. I felt reassured by this sight.

Then my mentor beckoned me to the nurses' desk and asked if I had seen a dead body before. I felt a bolt of shock – no, I hadn't. She took me to May's bedside. May was lying there very still. I was not prepared for her to be dead, and I could not believe it at first. How could she be dead when she still had her fluffy slippers on? It did not make any sense. I must have gone pale because the staff nurse suggested that I go and sit down and have a cup of tea. She was very kind.'

Reflective practice starts with a story like this one from our nurse training. Stories connect us. When people get together, they tell stories, and when nurses are with other nurses, they do the same. Through storytelling we find shared meanings about

---

Returning to Nursing Practice: Confidence and Competence, First Edition. Ros Wray and Mary Kitson.
© 2023 John Wiley & Sons Ltd. Published 2023 by John Wiley & Sons Ltd.

our lives. As Storr (2019) puts it: 'There's simply no way to understand the human world without stories.'

As nurses, we all have memorable recollections, narratives of significant events which have helped to shape our personal nursing history. We share our stories with each other because they serve to bond us together, helping us to de-brief, each re-telling adding another a layer of connection and reciprocity. Moon and Fowler (2008) call these 'known stories' because both tellers and listeners have in common an understanding of the experience of being a nurse. In Chapter 6 we will see how these shared narratives can help to strengthen our resilience when burdened with the emotional cost of caring for others. Bolton and Delderfield (2018, p. 84) say that as practitioners we tell our stories 'to take some of these incidents outside of ourselves' helping us to gain perspective and understanding about our feelings, thoughts and belief systems. As we move through one experience after another, we use our voices to come to know the nature of what we do and who we are (Oelofsen 2012; Duke 2013). Reflecting on our nursing work and taking forward new ideas and fresh learning, we perceive ourselves evolve. With growing self-awareness comes also sharpened critique and an increasing ability to see what might be beneath the surface of things. The first-year student nurse in the story just related learnt that day that death and fluffy slippers will often come together, that her innermost being will be shaken sometimes by what she witnesses, but that a good mentor will understand and offer comfort. The student went on to qualify, taking with her the memory of that critical day. The understanding of how much this kindness had mattered to her informed her future support for other students.

SELF-AWARENESS

'Knowing yourself is the beginning of all wisdom.'

– Aristotle.

Before we can truly make sense of our practice experiences, we must be self-aware. A key authority on the subject describes self-awareness as 'the continuous and evolving process of getting to know who you are' (Burnard 1992). Self-awareness is an important term in nursing, although you may not recall it featuring strongly in your original training. The concept has gained an integral place in nurse education over the last ten years with many contemporary university pre-registration nursing courses now centred on the development of the professional and personal self. Awareness of self and the impact we have on others fosters therapeutic relationships and nursing competence (Cook 2001; Rasheed 2015). In other words, the more we know of ourselves, the more we know how to care for others.

As you contemplate or embark on your return to nursing, you will know that you are not just updating knowledge and skills but also taking back a role. You will be activating a part of yourself which has been dormant. It is therefore a moment to revisit this professional nursing self and re-engage with what it means to you.

What do we mean by 'self'? The perception of self that relates to family may not be the same perception of self we have with friends on a night out. We share different parts of ourselves with different people. The roles we adopt in life mean that we develop and present varying aspects or versions of ourselves according to *context*. Burnard (1992) tells us that we have many selves: a private and public self, a physical and social self, a spiritual and emotional self, an ideal self, and of course a professional self. His publications contain a range of interesting activities designed to help us to further understand ourselves and are well worth reading.

There are a range of strategies to help us all enhance our self-awareness. Perhaps most famous is the Johari Window. First conceived in the mid-1950s, and still much in use today, this seminal resource comes in the form of an exercise designed to encourage self-insight. The name 'Johari' came from the names of those who created this model ('Jo' Luft and 'Harry' Ingham) and is shown in Figure 5.1.

The challenge of continually expanding our understanding of ourselves as nurses and individuals engages us all in lifelong learning (Jarvis 2010). The purpose of the exercise is to capture and reveal this forward movement and therefore to be of most benefit it needs to be repeated at regular intervals. As you find your way back to your nursing self, we recommend that you take some time to explore the Johari Window.

Pairing up with a trusted friend or family member, you are both asked to complete in stages the four quadrants. First complete the top left quadrant in the grid. This is the Open Area where you need to list things about yourself which you know, and others know too. For example, you might have brown eyes, be quite tall, and enjoy chocolate! Next, swap grids with your partner to complete the Blind Area. These are things which others know about you, but you may not. For example, your partner may write that you are inclined to hunch over your computer, give yourself too much to do in a day and leave doors open! Once digested, such revelations can be very helpful perhaps prompting a review of your working practices or maybe accounting for that neck stiffness in the late afternoons! With the grid back in your hands, you need now to turn your attention to the Hidden Area. Record here things which you know about yourself, but others may not. It is important to reveal only what you are happy

<table>
<tr><td></td><td></td><td colspan="2" align="center">Ask for feedback ⟶</td></tr>
<tr><td></td><td></td><td>Known to self</td><td>Not known to self</td></tr>
<tr><td rowspan="2">*Tell through self-disclosure*
↓</td><td>Known to others</td><td>Open Area</td><td>Blind Area</td></tr>
<tr><td>Not Known to others</td><td>Hidden Area</td><td>Unknown Area</td></tr>
</table>

FIGURE 5.1   The Johari Window. *Source:* Adapted from Luft and Ingham 1955.

now to share. For example, you may have always wanted to learn to sail, you may feel anxious about administering medicines again, and you may be frightened of frogs! Again, the grids are exchanged so that you can both see what the other has disclosed. Finally, it is time to consider the Unknown Area. This fourth quadrant looks to the future, charting those things unknown to you and others. As we come to see ourselves through feedback from others and through our own disclosures, we grow to understand ourselves more. What new things can you write here about yourself? What have you learnt through doing this exercise?

The processes of self-disclosure and feedback are dynamic and ongoing. Feedback during your return to nursing will be specific, issuing in the shape of comments on your practice and academic performance. You may find that some anxieties about writing assignments lighten when you discover with surprise that you still remember how to reference the literature. On the other hand, whilst acknowledging your empathetic approach with a patient, your Practice Assessor may also suggest that your time management skills require some attention, so delivering a message that may be uncomfortable to hear. Response to feedback can be emotional; however, this is often because it confronts an alternative view that we hold of ourselves. The Johari Window can work therapeutically helping us to acknowledge and validate these feelings, balancing our responses with the positive challenge of learning new things about ourselves.

As we become more comfortable with feedback our blind area shrinks and our self-knowledge expands. Similarly, our hidden area opens up as we self-disclose to others appropriately to show compassion and engender trust within our professional roles. Both feedback and self-disclosure help us towards a greater understanding of our unknown area. This bottom right quadrant in the grid is exciting because it holds understanding of our potential selves. It remains unknown to us today, but it will yield the insights of new growth and learning tomorrow, next year and into the future. In summary, the Johari Window stresses the significance of feedback and disclosure in relation to an ongoing and enhanced knowing of self.

Self-awareness paves the way to reflective practice. With growing insight into how and why we act and think as we do, we can start to reflect on our thoughts and feelings, our values and motivations, our assumptions, decisions and behaviours. We can come to understand more about the impact we have on others, the issues that affect us, and the way in which new experiences enable us to learn more about ourselves and other people in our daily and working lives. This ever-unfolding knowledge can help us to see things differently, and this can lead to change.

INTRODUCING REFLECTION

So, what does reflective practice mean to you? For some of you, it may be an unfamiliar or half-remembered concept, or you may recall it mainly as a form of assessment from your nurse training. Whatever your standpoint, we hope these discussions will offer a clear or refreshed perspective. If your thoughts do take you back to the sense of

an ever-present assignment which seemed to dog your nursing placements, the literature goes some way to agree, acknowledging that the use of reflective writing to assess
practice and academic competence is fraught with difficulty. Schutz (2013) points to
the sense of exposure which can be felt by students when asked for an honest expression of emotions which may then be judged within a summative assessment. She also
recognises that some of us may have the advantage of being more naturally adept at
reflecting than others. (This will be explained further in the next chapter when we
look at our individual personal learning styles.) There is no doubt that reflection is a
personal and complex activity which is often challenging. The act of reliving events
can be emotionally uncomfortable and intrusive, and yet since the 1980s reflective
practice has occupied a key place in nurse education (Mann et al. 2009; Jasper 2013).
Schutz (2013) concludes that this must be so because of its value in furthering our
understanding of nursing practice.

As we have already explained, returning to nursing will require you to be willing
and able to show others how you can reflect on and learn from your practice. Whether
this occurs as a verbal exchange or in written format, Bulman and Schutz (2013) highlight that it takes courage and open-mindedness to be able to receive and respond to
critical feedback from others. As the Johari Window demonstrates, the act of self-
disclosure through reflection brings risk and a sense of vulnerability. Bulman believes,
though, that we are driven as nurses to face these challenges because we are motivated constantly towards needing to know more about who we are as nurses, what we
do and how we can do it better. So, what is it about the activity of reflecting that makes
it so intrinsic to this endeavour? It is time to explore some underpinning theory.

DIPPING INTO THE THEORY!

Focus on learning through reflection is not exclusive to nursing. Students and practitioners throughout the professions (police, teaching, medicine and social work – to
name a few) are required to reflect on their practice to demonstrate their ongoing
development. Reflective practice has its own body of knowledge with published literature spanning the professions. It is crucial, therefore, to explore why reflective activity
is deemed so integral to professional learning. We are going to dip below the surface
of practice and practice learning to see what might be going on. Figure 5.2 helps to
provide a visual representation of these processes.

Reflection could be argued to be akin to a natural, almost automatic process of
mulling over something that has happened. It is a kind of mental sorting through
which feels necessary and often therapeutic for maintaining well-being. After a challenging day we all benefit from the chance to talk things over with someone we trust.
If we take this process and add in a structure and skills, we arrive at a reflective practice which helps us to examine complex experiences with a view to future learning.
This is an informing practice helping to make sense of what occurs everyday with the
potential to enable change. Like connecting threads between two edges of a garment,
reflective practice moves back and forth between nursing knowledge and nursing

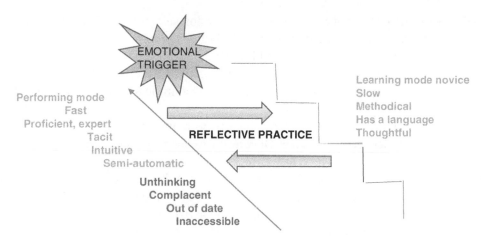

FIGURE 5.2 Reflective theory diagram. *Source:* Adapted and informed by understandings from Schon 1987; Benner 2001; Jarvis 2006; Eraut 2007.

action. Questions and points of learning bring together theory and practice, generating understandings of our own nursing experiences and fostering an ongoing spirit of inquiry.

We would like you to cast your minds back to your nurse training and ask you to recall how you learnt to administer an injection. How were you taught this skill? It is likely that the entire activity was broken down into stages which were methodical and graduated. As novices we tend to acquire skills step-by-step (represented by the steps in Figure 5.2). Procedures that need to be learnt are often presented to us in manageable pieces, so we can repeat and internalise each part before moving on to the next. These are the motor performance skills needed to deliver both comfort and safety in patient care (Baillie 2014). The Royal Marsden Manual of Clinical Procedures exemplifies this approach to learning with safe patient care enabled and represented by a series of standardised steps (Lister et al. 2020).

You may have practised your injection technique on a training device, or an orange or each other but, at some point, you will have progressed from repeating the action to assimilating this skill into your patient care. What happens to those steps of learning when you become good at giving injections? In the diagram you will see that opposite the steps there is a long diagonal arrow representing action that has become smooth and streamlined from repetition. As we rehearse the learning stages and absorb their guiding rules, we become more able to deliver a skilled performance (Eraut 2007). The procedure has been repeated and learnt many times and it can now be delivered again and again as needed. Our practice has become swift and proficient, giving that satisfying sense of flow which you may well remember from your previous nursing experience. It is worth pausing here for a moment to look at what is meant by 'flow'. A leading American psychologist, Csikszentmihalyi (2002), first coined the word 'flow' following research which revealed that people seem at their happiest when they are 'in the zone' or flow of an activity. If the activity brings sufficient challenge to engage but not over-tax, we can abandon self and time in a flow of intense focus which brings with it feelings of profound satisfaction.

We will explore Csikszentmihalyi's Flow Model further in a later chapter when we look at what helps to sustain our well-being and happiness. Here, though, flow is acknowledged as a component of competent performance. The immersion in action that characterises flow can bring with it a tacit outward state and one that feels semi-automatic: we know what we are doing and therefore there is no requirement for further comment, question or even deliberate thinking. Once you can swim or ride a bicycle, you do not need to think about how you do it anymore. Indeed, often to concentrate consciously on these actions, once internalised, is to sabotage them. Schon, a key writer on reflective practice, uses the term 'knowing-in-action' to describe the understanding required to ride a bicycle, pointing out that we are ill-equipped to verbalise this knowing to others even though we may be competent cyclists (Schon 1987). The knowing is hidden from view because it has become so embedded in action. Herein lies a potential problem.

As Figure 5.2 shows, and as we have outlined, this smooth flow of practice feels swift, efficient and rewarding to the practitioner, and indeed is necessary to carry out nursing work. However, could there be negative elements to this kind of practice? A practice that repeats itself semi-automatically can become unthinking, and therefore risks becoming out of date and drifting into complacency (Schon 1991; Jarvis 2006; Johns 2009).

Imagine that you are driving on your usual route from A to B. This is a very familiar journey and so whilst driving you are also pondering on your forthcoming weekend. You can drive proficiently and know the road well, so you do not have to focus on every signpost or turn in the road. Suddenly in front of you there is a big yellow diversion sign blocking the familiar road ahead and directing you down a road you have never been down before. How do you feel?

Emotions that burst through when things do not go according to plan are of great importance to reflective learning. Your response to the roadblock may range from annoyance and frustration to panic. One thing is clear, though – it is no longer possible to continue to think of other things. Emotional triggers interrupt that smooth, semi-automatic mode, the 'flow' characterised by the long arrow in Figure 5.2, forcing us to stop. This is crucial to reflective learning and is what Jarvis (2006) calls 'disjuncture'. Now we are in the moment, and this roadblock moment is an uncomfortable place where we will need to problem solve. We must take notice and work out a new route. The diagram shows how this change of thinking is sparked by an emotional trigger and leads back to a more thoughtful process which is step-by-step, slower more methodical. We are back to the learning mode mentioned earlier which, with its careful attention and steady pace, gives us the best chance of a good outcome in a new and uncertain situation. The process which enables us to learn from significant experiences is captured within reflective practice which encourages a questioning of what happened and a plan as to how to take the resulting learning forward. The arrows in the diagram represent that constant movement back and forth as we perform, learn, then perform again, ever developing new knowledge for practice through reflecting on our nursing experiences. This is an exciting dynamic which can lead to the discovery of new insights, uncovering fresh aspects of ourselves and adding to our personal knowing of our own nursing practice (Schon 1991; Dahlgren et al. 2004; Eraut 2007).

However, it can also be uncomfortable and challenging. When you return to nursing practice you are likely to start in step-by-step mode and therefore will need to have patience. Progress may feel slow. You will need to repeat and practise to build competence and confidence, and this will involve talking through and monitoring what you are doing very regularly. To go back to our earlier bicycle analogy, if your Practice Supervisor behaves like a professional cyclist performing silently and seamlessly, the only way to pierce this smooth outer skin of performance is to ask a question. Although practice is hard to articulate, questioning helps to slow things down, facilitating dialogue and the sharing of decision making. Additionally, as we have already identified, interrupting the flow of practice of others is important and necessary for their professional learning, guarding against complacency and resistance to change (Eraut 2007). Questions encourage joint reflection, enabling both student and supervisor to appreciate each other's viewpoint. Return to Practice students have much to share and as they retrieve their knowledge and skills, and feel encouraged to put forward ideas, a sense of collaboration and reciprocity between returner and supervisor very soon follows.

One returner recounted an experience from her placement which left her convinced of the fundamental necessity of adopting a questioning approach. Her practice setting was a secure unit for people with a learning disability. She had been encouraged by another nurse to assist a patient with autism to choose some new trainers, using a laptop and printer to make the order and provide her patient with a picture of what he had selected. When he asked repeatedly for one more printout, following a behavioural trait unknown to her, she was unable to oblige because of her limited access to the printer. Unfortunately, this triggered anxiety for the patient which escalated into a difficult episode. The student had to leave the area until the situation had been calmed. At first her feelings of guilt and disappointment about what had happened led to a sudden loss of confidence; she felt that if she had known more about the patient's behaviours, she would have been better prepared. Reflecting further on the event, she realised that both she and the nurse had assumed that the activity would be easy. The nurse had been keen to promote a positive experience and the student had responded with enthusiasm. The returner's future learning centred on the need to check and clarify even the most seemingly simple activities with the anticipatory question – 'Is there anything more I should be aware of?' She shared this idea with others on the unit, and the approach was readily adopted. Interactive discussions increased in the unit and the whole team subsequently became more reflective in their practice.

MODELS AND FRAMEWORKS AND THE REFLECTIVE PROCESS

Our roadblock analogy, albeit simplistic, has demonstrated the importance of recognising how the emotional dimension of an experience signals a cue for learning, and how crucial it is that we follow this trail. The need to reflect takes us to a more conscious awareness, urging us to take time out to think through what has happened. We must return to a learning mode which enables thoughtful problem solving and a language to articulate this activity. Over the years writers have developed models and frameworks designed to formulate this process. A step-by-step purposeful movement is encouraged that takes us from the story and feelings of an experience towards an understanding of its underlying meaning and significance and on to a point of fresh insight and potential change. These frameworks have been deliberately structured to slow our natural tendencies to seek quick answers, ensuring that we sit with the issues first, allowing time for processing and the surfacing of new ideas. This pacing can also have a therapeutic effect, allowing emotions to be voiced and then balanced proportionately.

Reflective models and frameworks guide us through these steps, varying slightly one from another in their respective forms and emphases, but all sharing the same basic reflective process. Jasper (2013), a key writer on reflective practice, calls this process Experience – Reflection – Action (ERA). Put simply, the experience is followed by thinking, reflecting and understanding it, and then moving forward with a new action plan. You will see this underlying process of reflection used in many areas of nursing including continuing professional development, collaborative debriefs, clinical supervision and the assessment of your competence during your return to practice placement.

Words of Wisdom

Using a reflective model was useful in giving structure to my writing but it also took me out of my comfort zone by making me consider my practice from angles that I might not ordinarily have done. If you struggle with one reflective model, I suggest trying different ones until you find one that works for you. When you become more confident, perhaps think about stepping outside your comfort zone with a model that makes you question your practice in a new way.

This student has already started to explore different models, realising that each has something individual to offer. Many practitioners go on to develop their own framework for reflecting on their practice. Below we have outlined two established frameworks with examples to show you how they work. There are many more to discover which you will find outlined in the literature (Bulman and Schutz 2013; Jasper 2013; Howatson-Jones 2016).

BORTON (1970) AND DRISCOLL (1994, 2007)

Figure 5.3 shows an amalgamation of Borton's (1970) and Driscoll's reflective structures (1994, 2007). What? So What? Now What? This is a simple three-stage framework which perhaps offers less structure but more flexibility. Cue questions have been suggested within each phase to aid reflective thinking; we must also here acknowledge the work of Rolfe et al. (2001) who have developed this structure to accentuate the Now What? part of the process, highlighting that the spiral of continuing learning mentioned earlier is also a spiral of action and change. Later in this chapter we will

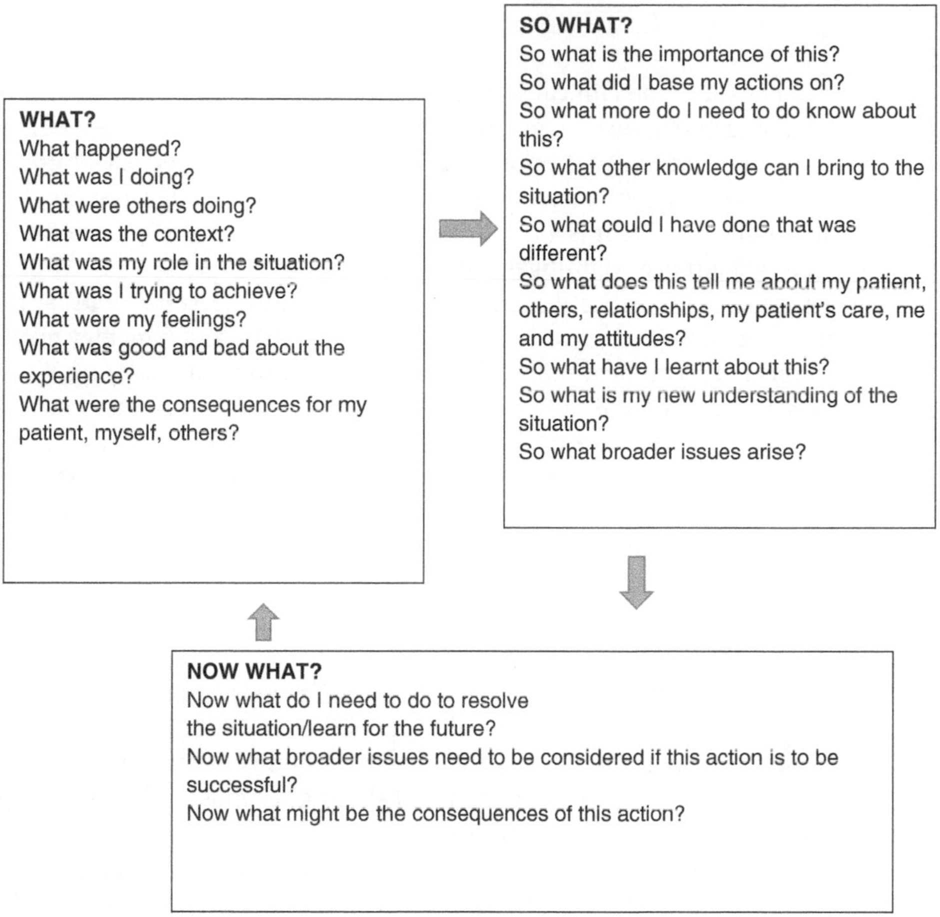

SO WHAT?
So what is the importance of this?
So what did I base my actions on?
So what more do I need to do know about this?
So what other knowledge can I bring to the situation?
So what could I have done that was different?
So what does this tell me about my patient, others, relationships, my patient's care, me and my attitudes?
So what have I learnt about this?
So what is my new understanding of the situation?
So what broader issues arise?

WHAT?
What happened?
What was I doing?
What were others doing?
What was the context?
What was my role in the situation?
What was I trying to achieve?
What were my feelings?
What was good and bad about the experience?
What were the consequences for my patient, myself, others?

NOW WHAT?
Now what do I need to do to resolve the situation/learn for the future?
Now what broader issues need to be considered if this action is to be successful?
Now what might be the consequences of this action?

FIGURE 5.3   Borton (1970) and Driscoll (1994, 2007) combined reflective model. *Source:* Adapted from Borton (1970) & Driscoll (1994 & 2007).

show how a student was able to use this framework to transform her practice, taking note of and researching tiny but significant details about her patient which had at first gone unnoticed.

REFLECTIVE THINKING AND WRITING SKILLS

As already stated, some Return to Practice courses ask very little in terms of academic assessment, concentrating almost entirely on practice. Other courses will involve submission of academic work. However, whichever course you opt for, to meet NMC standards for registered nurses, you will need to demonstrate your ability to reflect on your nursing practice, both verbally and in a written format (NMC 2016). These are specific skills which you will be able to develop or retrieve as you progress.

Observing

Your first steps back into the clinical setting are likely to be directed towards observing, re-acclimatising and adjusting, and this is as it should be. These understandable and necessary drivers naturally take precedence until you have settled back into practice and can take stock of your surroundings. Of these three activities, observation is key. The ability to be observant is a universally acknowledged nursing attribute perhaps first noted by Florence Nightingale who wrote in 1860:

'The most important practical lesson that can be given to nurses is to teach them what to observe (and) how to observe' (Nightingale 1969, p. 105). Although they may feel latent, your clinical observational skills will be well honed from years of nurse training and experience. These same skills of looking, hearing and sensing are prerequisites for reflection because, as we have already set out, reflective practice starts with the recalling of experience. Many who write about reflection place emphasis on this first step. One such writer is Johns (2009) who, known for his focus on self-expression, encourages us to use all five senses to capture the richness of the story part of the experience.

Keeping a Diary

A good place to record your observations is in a diary. There is evidence to show that the act of writing engages the brain in thinking (Boud et al. 1985; Heron and Corradini 2020). As you capture the detail of experience your mind is sifting and picking up on strands and cues, making connections and asking questions which will help to uncover the meanings of what has occurred.

Diaries and journals come in many forms. Whether purely a list of things to do, or a personal journey of thoughts and ideas, the keeping of a diary may be something that you have already found of value. At its most basic level, the written word provides an aide memoire, preserving the tiny details of an experience which might otherwise have been forgotten. Our memories of events can alter over time. We might unconsciously select and heighten certain elements because they fit our expectations and viewpoints and allow other less accommodating aspects to fade. The passage of time too plays its part, often dimming events so that only what felt significant is remembered. Therefore, the capturing of detail soon after an experience is vital to reflective practice because it gives us the best chance of recording things as they truly occurred.

Words of Wisdom

During my placement I kept a journal. It is the best thing I could have done. I did not worry too much about using a particular model when writing it but maintaining the journal was helpful, both as a means of off-loading after a difficult shift but also because I had forgotten a lot of what happened on placement when it came to reflective writing. When I read through my journal, I realised I had been reflecting all along!

In practical terms, you will need to decide on the format of your diary. For those of us who prefer to use pen and paper the attraction of selecting a new piece of stationery is hard to resist! Others may gravitate to a Word document or even an audio file. Whatever your medium, crucial to sustaining a diary is getting this choice right so that you feel at one with the activity. Return to Practice courses are unlikely to require you to record your experiences in this way, and we are not suggesting that you embark on pages and pages of effort. Jack and Smith (2007) encourage us to use our own short-hand codes so that the activity feels manageable and meaningful. This builds on the work of earlier influential writers, Boud et al. (1985), who place feelings at the heart of our reflective practice and urge that these be expressed honestly. For them, maintaining a journal is vital to reflective learning, and they recommend we set aside time for it. Tate (2013) agrees, portraying the act of keeping a diary as one of purpose and commitment. In their raw form of course, diaries and journals are considered private; however, they will provide you with source material on which to base shared writing such as course assignments.

A good tip is to keep your notes to one page or section with space nearby to add later thoughts. Early observations and descriptions will lead on to deeper thinking and ideas and it is useful to be able to link the two together. Diary-keeping can reveal patterns in your thinking, beliefs and assumptions which you might not otherwise have seen (Tate 2013; Bolton and Delderfield 2018). These insights may lead you to think anew about current experiences and your future actions.

Often the most significant areas of learning lie hidden in what might first seem inconsequential. For example, our respective efforts to keep a journal during the coronavirus pandemic seemed to consist in a faithful and sometimes obsessive cataloguing of facts and figures; indeed, these do provide an accurate record. However, on re-reading, what is most striking are the personal reflections on how it felt to be in lockdown. Comfort came from little things: a walk during late January, sparkling with snow and full of the shriek of children sledging; the appearance of a wren pertly sorting out old autumn leaves; an unexpected text from a school friend sharing her photo of a glowing sunset. During those strange times, we learnt that well-being meant still feeling connected. It meant keeping the senses alive. The necessity and pleasure of daily exercise, the sounds and smells of a beautiful summer and warm communication with loved ones took on heightened importance. We will return to some of these ideas in our chapter on well-being. Of chief concern here is the process of capturing our observations. From such descriptive details and stories come underlying themes and meanings.

DESCRIBING

We started this chapter with the importance of storytelling, and we have also seen that keeping a diary can capture key moments. Academic reflective writing rightly places emphasis on analysis because of course this is where deeper meanings and significant insights come to the surface, informing future practice. However, the reflective process demands first a description of the event or experience, and this is vital.

Descriptive language has the power to communicate and evoke, in itself enhancing a shared understanding of what we do (Benner 2001); and without the rich detail of the story, a full critique cannot happen. Each experience is rendered unique by the people, contexts, timeframes and occurrences involved; the analysis that follows, therefore, is shaped by these details. Duke (2013) also urges us to value our descriptions of practice, concerned that we safeguard our individual nursing voice seen reflected in the story of our own individual experience. Whilst formal in its style and structure, academic reflective writing preserves the voice of the writer through the use of the first person; this is unlike traditional academic work where objectivity is reinforced by writing in the third person. The examples below come from an overseas nurse as she begins to learn about practice in a nursing home placement. Example 1 shows her first attempt to tell her story. In the second we see how she was able to revise her work with support from her personal tutor and using Borton & Driscoll's reflective model of What? So What? Now What?

EXAMPLE 1

Mr. T was an eighty-four-year-old gentleman with Parkinson's Disease. He was unable to weight bear and needed much help with all his personal hygiene. I was working in the morning with a Healthcare Assistant, and we were helping Mr. T to get up. We had helped him to wash and dress and we needed to transfer him from the bed to his chair. We got the hoist and placed the sling around him and connected it up to the hooks. However, when we started to lift him up using the hoist he seemed to slip in the sling, and he became distressed. I felt terrible thinking that he was going to fall out of the sling. We quickly lowered him back on to the bed. Although I believed that I had followed the correct procedure for using the hoist, this experience has made me realise that I need to redo my moving and handling training as I must have done something wrong.

EXAMPLE 2

What? – Description

Mr. T was an eighty-four-year-old tall gentleman who was suffering with Parkinson's Disease. His condition made his movements slow and jerky and his joints were quite stiff. He was unable to weight bear and needed much help with all his personal hygiene. I was working in the morning with a Healthcare Assistant, and we were helping Mr. T to get up. We had helped him to wash and dress and we needed to transfer him from the bed to his chair. Having explained to him what we needed to do and received his consent, we got the hoist and placed the sling around him as he lay on the bed. We connected the hooks to the hoist. However, as we started to lift him up using the hoist he seemed to slip in the sling, and he became distressed. I felt terrible thinking that he was going to fall out of the sling. We quickly lowered him back on to the bed.

So What? – Analysis

I knew that we had both followed the correct procedure for using the hoist. However, something had gone wrong. I thought about Mr. T and how shaky and stiff he was and remembered that it had been challenging to get the sling into the right position. Mr. T was a very tall man who found it difficult to move his joints. Sufferers of Parkinson's Disease often experience rigidity and cannot move quickly (NICE 2017). Although we had obtained consent and followed our moving and handling training, his stiffness and slow movements meant that he was sitting in an awkward position in the sling and therefore this jolted him when we lifted him up. We had moved him too quickly. The European Parkinson's Disease Association (EPDA 2016) states the importance of taking time when looking after patients with Parkinson's Disease.

Now What? – Future Action

In the future I will remember to take time when looking after a patient with Parkinson's Disease. I will need to read more about how the condition specifically affects movement so that I can use the hoist more carefully and in a way that promotes dignity and ensures patient safety and comfort.

Here we are reminded of the importance of a carefully recounted description (Bolton and Delderfield 2018). The small descriptive details about Mr. T's height and stiff joints determined the direction of the analysis. The resulting learning and action were not about needing to redo moving and handling training; the point of analysis is finely tuned to the individual nurse and the individual patient.

CHOOSING YOUR EXPERIENCE

The notion that we choose an experience is misleading and probably comes from the way in which students are often required to seek out a suitable practice experience to reflect on for the purposes of completing an academic assignment. Whilst this is often a required element of assessment of professional education, and not without contention (Johns 2009; Schutz 2013), the reality is that the experience usually chooses us. In their early seminal paper, Atkins and Murphy (1993) refer to the way in which problematic experiences can leave us with uncomfortable feelings which niggle, telling us that there is something more to understand. Such emotions act as a signal, urging us to look more closely, motivating us towards new learning. In the above illustration, the student says that 'she felt terrible'. Her sense of dismay and self-blame is palpable. It is this that has sparked the reflection. Whilst reflective inquiry is more likely to be triggered by difficult or challenging events, sometimes positive feelings of surprise or delight can also initiate the process. We remember a nursing student who could not contain her sense of wonder on witnessing a water birth during her community placement. She reflected on the intuitive actions of the midwife who listened and responded to the needs of the soon-to-be Mum, sharing the joyful anticipation of the family as she gauged the water temperature. This led the student to further research water births so that she could understand how the midwife had been able to almost invisibly balance safe clinical judgement with the nurturing of a calm and homely atmosphere. She learnt about the science of water immersion in labour and the 'professional artistry' of expert midwifes (Schon 1987). Schon is one of the forefathers of reflection and has much to say about the attributes of reflective practitioners; we will look at his work in a little more detail towards the end of the chapter.

When it comes to reflective writing for assignment purposes, choosing the right experience is a skill. Perhaps more than any other, critical incidents and emergencies require reflective analysis. However, these events are often too complex and large-scale to manage within the confines of a short reflective account. You may feel drawn to such momentous experiences because they carry an emotional charge and involve many people. However, this kind of reflection is best managed as a group activity or as part of clinical supervision with the aim of facilitating collaborative learning and therapeutic debriefing in a practice context. For reflective assignments it is important to select an event that has discrete boundaries in terms of size and scope. Final assessments usually have a specified word count and are concerned with an individual's practice learning. They require a clear focus on a single event usually related to patient care. Sometimes assignment guidelines will direct you further, requiring that the experience you select demonstrates a particular skill or topic such as health promotion or leadership.

GIBBS REFLECTIVE CYCLE (1988)

This model is one of the most well-known. It connects strongly to experiential learning theory, drawing on the work of Kolb (1984), an earlier educational theorist. The reflective cycle is shown in Figure 5.4 and is accompanied by a summary of each of the six stages.

Description

Gibbs first stage requires us to describe what happened. Capturing with clarity the details of the event in this way is vital, so we need to choose our language carefully so that it paints an accurate picture. This is the what, where, when and who of the story and, importantly, we must relate here the full and complete experience. Whatever is in the story is then analysed at a later point; if the narrative is not contained in this first section, but continues to trickle out through the remaining cycle, it will water down the structure and dilute the analysis, making it hard to delve to uncover underlying themes.

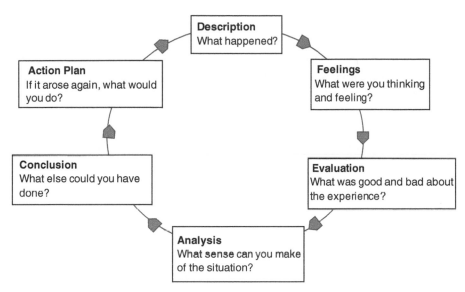

FIGURE 5.4   Gibbs reflective cycle. *Source:* Modified from Gibbs G (1988).

Thoughts and Feelings

Often, meaningful experience engages us first at an emotional level. We have seen earlier how strong feelings trigger the urge to reflect because we have a need to understand what has taken place. Emotions drive the analysis and fasten to the learning. As Jarvis puts it: 'we do learn from and through our feelings' (2006, p. 6). It is crucial, therefore, that we try to find the right words to accurately and honestly express how we feel about an experience, although this may be elusive and difficult straight after the event. Precise vocabulary such as 'awkward', 'proud', 'frustrated' or 'embarrassed' should be used and acknowledged so that the lines of inquiry during the analysis are directed towards relevant learning. It is also helpful at this stage to try to think about the thoughts and feelings of others in the experience.

Words of Wisdom

Reflective practice can be uncomfortable. Reflection is often triggered by emotion and can feel challenging to write because so much of our working day is about documenting what we have done or plan to do with or for our patients and we are told to write about the facts. Reflective practice is much more about how **we** are feeling and not all of us feel at home writing about ourselves! I found discussing my topic with tutors and peers helpful because we were all going through similar experiences.

Evaluation

This third stage marks a transition from what has been individual, subjective and descriptive to something more objective; this prepares us for the analysis. We are asked to consider what did not go well, and what did go well, levelling out our emotional response to enable a greater range of perspective. This shift in gear shows how the cycle can also work therapeutically, as here what might have seemed a negative experience starts to feel more positive. Bolton and Delderfield (2018) rationalise this apparent contradiction by explaining that reflective writing provides the medium to both connect us to and distance us from the experience.

Analysis

Analysis is about asking questions of something whole so that it can be broken down into its constituent parts. What do we need to explore to further understand? Here we are looking at the why (in all its forms) of the experience. Why did I feel the way I did? What informed the patient's decision making? Why was the relative asking so many questions? We arrive at the themes and factors underlying the experience and these become lines of investigation, taking us to the literature. Bulman and Schutz (2013) caution us to concentrate only on key priorities so that the analysis does not stretch superficially but has critical depth.

Conclusion

This fifth stage draws together our findings. What was the learning gained from the experience? Armed with new insight, we ask what could have been done differently. Alternative approaches may swing into view.

Action Plan

We are now set to move forward with a clear idea of what we would do differently next time. This last stage takes our learning from one experience into the future with a specific plan of action. Although Gibbs cycle appears closed, the intention is that we move on in a kind of spiral, each new practice encounter or situation informed by what has gone before. Thus, we engage in ongoing professional development with the potential to perform with greater knowledge, skills and understanding.

The following is an example of a reflective assignment written by one of our returning students using Gibbs reflective cycle. The references used in the account have been added to the list at the end of the chapter.

Returner's account

Description

I introduced myself to Mrs. F and helped the staff nurse to settle her ready for her morning medication. This patient was 77 years old and was suffering with advanced dementia. She had a Deprivation of Liberty Safeguard (DoLS) under the Mental Capacity Act 2005 which allowed other people to make decisions in her best interests. I was about to leave when the staff nurse tried to administer oral medication to Mrs. F. At this point things became problematic. Mrs. F was very resistant, clenching her teeth and hitting out at the staff nurse. At first, I felt unable to respond. Cautiously, I asked the nurse if she would like me to try and she said 'yes', confiding that she was finding it difficult.

I drew the curtains to ensure privacy and prevent distractions. I was aware that we had both been standing up and this could appear threatening, so I asked the staff nurse to sit down (explaining it would take a while, so I did not seem too bossy). I sat down close to Mrs. F so that she could see my face. Then speaking slowly and clearly, I reintroduced myself, giving Mrs. F time to process (National Health Service 2020.) Although Mrs. F did not have a hearing aid, I was aware that people over seventy often have some degree of hearing loss, so I made sure that my voice was calm but slightly louder (McNamara 2016). I tentatively reached out my hand which she took, and which seemed to confirm that she was composed. I explained that there was medicine that the doctor wanted her to take. I gave her time to process this information. Then I gently helped her to take her medication, ensuring that the medicine pot was visible. I used short sentences, spoke softly and ensured that we took pauses so that she did not feel rushed. As she slowly drank the medicine, I adjusted the angle of the medicine pot so that she felt in control and was safe from choking or aspiration. With each sip I reassured her and in a relatively short space of time all the medicine was gone. Mrs. F had remaining calm and comfortable throughout.

Afterwards the staff nurse commented on how easy it had seemed. We took time to reflect on what had happened, and I shared my recent experience working in a dementia care home. I had also attended a dementia awareness course which had focused on advanced communication skills. The staff nurse told me that it was difficult not to rush on a busy acute ward, but that this experience had reminded her to be sufficiently self-aware to be able to slow down.

Thoughts and Feelings

This was a challenging situation for me. I felt concerned when the patient became upset, and I knew that I possessed the skills and understanding to alleviate her distress. At the same time, the staff nurse was in charge, and I felt very hesitant about intervening. However, as things worsened, the nurse looked at me and I realised that she needed my help. I knew that she felt embarrassed and was pleased that I found a way to act tactfully with consideration of her feelings. I think it took courage for the staff nurse to admit that she needed assistance, and this in turn gave me the confidence to step forward.

Evaluation

Communicating with patients suffering with dementia can be very challenging. Unfortunately, Mrs. F had become unnecessarily distressed because she had felt rushed and pressured. My student status and lack of confidence led me to hesitate. However, on a more positive note, I was eventually able to calm Mrs. F so that she could take her medication. I used skilled communication techniques and was also able to sustain good relations with the staff nurse. We both benefited from discussing the incident afterwards.

Analysis

It was crucial that I upheld Mrs. F's dignity and treated her as an individual. Her DoLS status required me to act in her best interests, offering person-centred care and taking responsibility for her safety (NMC 2018). I know that people with dementia can have slower thought processing and therefore it was important not to rush (McNamara 2016). My prior experience helped me to feel confident and this relaxed my body language, a significant factor in communicating with dementia patients (McNamara 2016).

Dementia causes a decline in cognitive functioning and language skills. Williams et al. (2009) use the term 'physical resistiveness to care' to describe the non-verbal responses of people with dementia which can include clenching teeth, turning away and holding arms close to the body. Mrs. F was displaying these signs. It has been suggested that a tone of voice which conveys a level of control can trigger resistiveness to care (Williams and Herman 2011). The staff nurse had been standing over Mrs. F and her voice had grown more instructive, and this seemed to correlate with Mrs. F's increasing distress. Her resistiveness to care was her way of saying no. As much as 90% of communication with people with advanced dementia is non-verbal (McNamara 2016). Meaningful communication with those at the more advanced stages of dementia remains very challenging and requires a high level of competence (Downs and Bowers 2008; De Vries 2013). In addition, Bridges and Wilkinson (2011) suggest that many nurses do not feel confident about negotiating with someone who does not want to take their medication.

The reflective debrief with the staff nurse affirmed my competence. Her honest response also taught me the importance of supportive teamwork, and the importance of acknowledging to others when things are challenging.

Conclusion

This experience highlighted the extent to which busy acute environments can feel stressful and alarming, especially for those suffering with dementia. Competing priorities and heavy workloads can result in key communication skills becoming compromised. The importance of taking time, awareness of body language and tone of voice, and an understanding of advanced dementia enabled me to promote the well-being of a vulnerable patient, whilst retaining her dignity (Scriven 2017). I could have acted sooner if I had felt more confident; however, the situation felt positive because it led to a reflective conversation during which both gained new learning.

Action Plan

This experience boosted my self-confidence and affirmed my ability to communicate well with dementia patients. I have learnt the value of my past knowledge and skills. In a similar future situation, I could now take the lead and act as an effective role model. Following our discussion, the staff nurse encouraged me to plan a teaching session on advanced communication with dementia patients for other students and staff members. This will help to raise awareness in a busy clinical setting and enable me to further my own understanding.

The stages of Gibbs reflective cycle helped me to unpick this experience (Gibbs 1988). The process of analysis enabled me to question what happened, appreciate differing perspectives and reach new insights about the challenges of caring for someone with advanced dementia in a fast-paced acute clinical setting. I have learnt the value of reflective dialogue with other practitioners; this was only made possible because the staff nurse was willing to disclose to me how she felt. Her example has encouraged me to explore this area in future practice.

Here we see how an honest appeal from a busy staff nurse emboldens a returner to intervene. Again, the description stage preserves the tiny key details of the returner's skilled intervention, preparing the later points of analysis where the returner's examination of the literature reinforces her understandings of advanced dementia, strengthening her evidence base for practice.

Her initial thoughts and feelings are also crucial to note. The returner moves from hesitancy to concern for the patient to feeling the nurse's discomfort to reaching the confidence to act. This interplay of thought and emotion tells of the uncertainty and complexity of exercising authority in a student role. It is of course not always possible to fully understand a patient's perspective, and, in this example, it must have been especially difficult. Nonetheless, we sense her personal values of empathy and compassion as she observes what is happening. Her decision to take the lead reveals an eventual recognition of herself as an experienced and skilled practitioner who is needed. The situation happened to one individual; however, the underlying themes echo the seesawing of confidence and competence commonly felt by many returning nurses.

ANALYSING

Analysis is often seen as the most important stage of the reflective process because it connects story to meaning (Rolfe et al. 2011; Duke 2013). Through the asking of questions, we can move from description to critique, from the individual to the universal, from subjective emotion to a more objective reasoning.

Finding the Evidence Base

We see in the returner's reflective piece that she has searched the literature concerned with advanced dementia to find the precise sources which will evidence her discussion on physical resistiveness to care. Pinpointing the exact concept or line of inquiry is crucial in reflective analysis because it is this that makes sense to the eventual learning and any future action. However, supporting reflective writing with the appropriate evidence base can be tricky and elusive. The nature of some required underpinning can be so concrete and tangible that it may jump out at you. For example, if you have been examining the effect of dehydration on the skin, you may immediately reach for a reference to the relevant pathophysiology. However, other knowledge bases are harder to spot because they are abstract or link to softer skills such as communication. Here, the returner's prior experience gave her a confidence which resulted in a relaxed body language – something so subtle that it may not seem to warrant referencing; however, her self-awareness that this was a factor which enabled her to communicate with the patient is fundamental to helping her to find the courage to intervene. The literature on non-verbal communication in nursing is vast because these skills are central to our everyday practice and often highly developed.

Building Practice Knowledge

The simple questioning of an experience helps us to see beneath the surface. We begin to discover other viewpoints and, crucially, some sense of the patient's experience when we learn in the above account how subtle changes in tone of voice can calm distress. Thinking through what each nurse might ask uncovers further meaning. The staff nurse may want to know how the returner was able to coax Mrs. F to take the medication. She may want to question why she found communicating with Mrs. F so challenging – What was I doing that triggered the patient's initial response? Why did I find it all so difficult? The returner may be pondering her delayed response, and how to support the staff nurse further in a way that is not awkward. Critical reflection involves considered and systematic self-questioning which has the potential to lead to a new knowing of practice and of ourselves as practitioners (Rolfe et al. 2011). Rolfe et al. (2011) explain how analysis of our individual experiences generates a personalised evidence base, or practice knowledge, which informs our future nursing work; knowing and doing loop together, becoming part of the same circle. An earlier collaborative research inquiry carried out by Higgs and Titchen (2001) shows how reflective interaction with colleagues can spark fresh insights into the nature of our professional practice. Clearly both participants have new knowledge to gain from this encounter.

Uncovering Assumptions

When we are able to look at all the angles of an experience, we become more aware of not just what, but how, we are thinking. With surprise we may suddenly grasp something that has been hidden from view. An important earlier theorist calls this moment 'perspective transformation' (Mezirow 2000). The returning nurse seems to experience such a moment when she suddenly realises that the staff nurse is struggling and needs her help. This shift in perspective flashes before her, propelling her to take the lead and overriding feelings of self-doubt. Such 'reflection-in-action' (Schon 1987) often steers us out and away from a fixed inner stance to a more open position of understanding. The staff nurse appears also to be caught in a set pattern of behaviour, interrupted only by the patient's protests. Brookfield (2012), a major proponent of critical thinking, warns us to be mindful of views based on generalised beliefs, assumptions or stereotypical thinking. An assumption is defined as 'a willingness to accept something as true without question or proof' (Cambridge English Dictionary 2022). We assume things all the time based on trust, past experience or habit, and often this is necessary and justified; for example, when we go to the supermarket it is reasonable to assume that shopping trolleys will be available for us to use. The underlying assumptions in the account may be that the returner must perform as a student and the staff nurse knows what she is doing. The reality may be more about one nurse struggling to balance a heavy workload with the needs of an agitated patient, and the other nurse able to support and bring resolution but apprehensive because of her student status.

To enable us to scrutinise our perspectives, Brookfield (2009) encourages to pose questions, checking to see what we might be overlooking or taking for granted. When the two nurses reflect together after the incident, a deeper level of understanding is reached. The staff nurse knew how to communicate with an individual suffering with dementia, so where and why did it all go wrong? Had she assumed that this knowledge would click into action? Why was the returner able to stay calm and unrushed? In learning mode was she more mindful than the staff nurse for whom, perhaps, drug administration had become too much of a standardised task? Did the returner assume that the staff nurse would not welcome her intervention? Was the staff nurse aware of the student's apprehension?

Thinking Time

> 'Time and reflection modify our vision, moreover, and at last we reach understanding.'
>
> (Cezanne in Danchev 2016)

Reflective analysis responds well to the passing of time. Like a good wine or cheese, our thinking matures when it is left to itself for a while. Often our human inclination is to move away as quickly as possible from uncomfortable feelings towards answers or actions that seems to offer comfort or resolution. Gibbs cautions against this haste to solve problems, explaining that it can shut down our critiquing processes too soon (Gibbs 1988). Any analysis that takes place straight after an event is likely to be on the thin side, often one-dimensional, a response to initial impressions and still encumbered with some residual emotion. Brookfield agrees, advocating the need for 'reflective pauses and interludes' – breaks in conscious focus which allow different perspectives to come to the surface (Brookfield 2012, p. 182). In the returner's account we can see key themes coming to the fore, including the need to develop finely tuned communication skills when caring for dementia patients in acute environments, and how courage exercised through honesty and assertiveness can lead to important shared learning. Of course, other deeper realisations may still emerge. In reality, significant events do not leave us; they continue to unfold quietly in the background, taking more meaningful shapes as we read around the topics concerned and discuss related ideas with others.

Words of Wisdom

I was glad I had allowed enough time to write the analysis – leave it for a while and come back to it. It enabled me to process the events and review my writing more objectively. I also realised there was no substitute for background reading. Once the main themes of my reflection had emerged, I read articles and book chapters which allowed me to add all the necessary references as I was writing. My advice: as long as you have lots of experiences from practice, the reflection will come – (most) nurses do it instinctively!

FUTURE LEARNING AND ACTION

This account exemplifies how the reflective process can affirm new insights and action for two individuals. In the face of difficulty, honest self-disclosure from the staff nurse has paused her practice giving her time to see afresh what might have drifted into an unthinking approach. It has also enabled the returner to feel that her prior knowledge and skills are needed. She learns the importance of being assertive and experiences a surge of confidence and competence. Supported by the staff nurse, the returner's plan of action is concrete and specific, and will hopefully help to raise awareness of advanced communication skills when caring for those with dementia.

Sometimes reflective practice can have an even broader reach, resulting in organisational change. We remember one student who noticed a client with severe learning disabilities would always closely observe when staff made him a cup of tea. The student deduced that perhaps the client wanted to make his own tea. Further inquiry with the team made it clear that this was thought too risky to try because the client tended to put everything into his mouth, including teabags. The student persisted. He went through the process of tea making with the client and each time the tea bag ended up in the client's mouth. Then one day, the client put the tea bag straight into the mug. A few days later he had learnt to make his own tea safely. This small and simple act made others think again about their approach to clients, sparking a shift in culture throughout the entire organisation. Collective assumptions about what individuals could and could not do were thrown open, resulting in transformative learning and new ways of caring. Learning at this deeper level can involve a critique and reorganisation of entire environments and systems of thinking (O'Sullivan et al. 2016). In our current post-pandemic climate, it could be argued that there is urgent need for healthcare professionals to feel part of a critically reflective and nurturing culture. As Kolb tells us: 'Learning is the process whereby knowledge is created through the transformation of experience' (1984, p. 38). Unfortunately, short-staffing and work pressures can mean that this is not always possible. However, Barchard (2021) reminds us of the advent of the professional nurse advocate role in England, introduced to provide nurses with the opportunity to pause, reflect and be supported and listened to (NHS 2021).

BEING A REFLECTIVE PRACTITIONER

Benner reminds us that nurses' stories illustrate the truth that their practice continually grows and develops through time and experience (Benner 2001). Every three years following your re-registration you will be required to complete your NMC

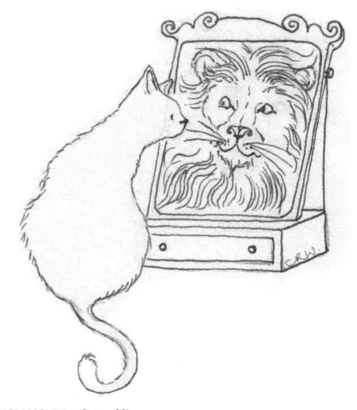

ILLUSTRATION NO. 5.1   Cat and lion.

professional revalidation, part of which asks you to compile five reflective accounts which demonstrate your compliance with the Code and your ongoing professional development (Nursing and Midwifery Council 2016). A verifier will confirm these activities by engaging in a meaningful reflective discussion about your practice learning and future objectives. Returning to nursing, therefore, is not just about updating clinical competencies but also about being a reflective practitioner.

Schon (1987) envisaged professional practice as the 'swampy lowlands'. Every step of a nursing day can sink into messy uncertainties and complexities. Yet nurses come to know and cherish the fact that this defines what they do. Many engage actively in reflection, exchanging new ideas with those around them. We believe that nurses returning to their profession are especially well-placed to inspire and encourage others, embracing the qualities that Schon attributes to the reflective practitioner. Returners have paused their practice. They have had time to reflect and often come back to the profession with insight matured from other life events. Reflective practitioners are described as possessing a store of remembered experiences which they draw on in their decision-making (Atkins and Schutz 2013). Informed by the learning from each unique encounter, they move forward, learning as they go, prepared to challenge rules that do not fit and be innovative in their problem-solving. The practice nurse returner who knew that her patient's wound should be reviewed daily to promote healing, also understood that omitting the dressing change for one day so that he could attend a family event was more beneficial to his overall well-being. Similarly, the palliative care nurse returner knew that whilst evidence-based practice seeks to reduce infection risks, her immune-compromised patient needed a catheter to ease the constant discomfort of skin soreness due to incontinence. Both nurses were able to reflect and justify to others how and why they made these complicated decisions.

Reflective practitioners are thought to exhibit a professional artistry, able to find a creative response to a perceived need (Schon 1987). These are often small finely observed acts such as re-positioning a bed by a window to lift the isolation felt by a non-English-speaking patient or ensuring that a stroke patient can get outside for a breath of fresh air to ease long days of intensive rehabilitation. These are the simple things which can make all the difference.

Reflective practice helps us to generate a living edge of inquiry. It connects emotion to learning and learning to change. We would like to end this chapter as we began – with a story. We are very grateful for this contribution from a former returning student who found reflective writing helpful in the face of personal loss. Her words take us beyond the course to the knowledge that for many of us, reflection can bring sense and meaning to a challenging world.

Words of Wisdom

During my nurse training back in the 1990s, 'reflective practice' was quite a 'buzz' term. My cohorts had to use reflection in our essay accounts. We were also encouraged to regard reflective practice as a way qualified nurses could learn from their experiences and develop their practice as a result. Returning to practice 25 years later, I was amazed that the concept of reflective practice was still very much on the nurse education agenda. Indeed, we were asked to write a reflective account. Though it had been a long time since I had written in this way, I felt that this would be a simple enough challenge.

However, the incident I choose to reflect upon created challenges that were initially quite uncomfortable. I had been widowed just a few months earlier and the incident I was reflecting on involved a dying patient of a similar age to myself. I choose to use a framework for reflection created by Borton (1970). This was not a framework I had used in my nurse training but was one that really appealed to me because of its quite straightforward approach. It asked me to consider 'What Happened', 'So What' and 'Now What'.

Using this model, I was able to constructively think about 'What Happened'. 'So What' had me considering more than just my initial feelings about the incident. At first, I had paid attention to the physical aspects of not having a quiet room for families needing support or space. Using the framework, I felt safe to explore the deeper issues around the incident and my own grief which felt quite raw and open again, as a result. Borton's framework gave me the space to consider the consequences of my own coping mechanisms and it allowed me to recognise the concept of 'burn out' helping me to see that I was at risk of 'burn out'. Through the reflection process I gained insight into how I had been bottling up my own grief and trying to busy myself as a way of avoiding it. Perceiving this, I spent hours researching the long-term effects of bottling up grief. These were not good, and I saw that I could be at a high risk of burn-out with my research also revealing that doctors and nurses are at a higher risk of burn-out because of their jobs. 'Now What' provided me with the prompt to look at what I could do pro-actively to reduce the chance of me suffering burn-out too. I recognised that I need to continue to work on my self-awareness and emotional intelligence.

Revisiting reflective practice as a part of my RTP course has really helped me as a registered nurse. I no longer consider my reflective practice as superficially as I had previously. I now view what a situation or incident means to my patient and what it means to me and my practice. Very importantly it encourages me to proactively think 'Now What' do I need to do about it.

REFERENCES

Atkins, S. and Murphy, C. (1993). Reflection: a review of the literature. *Journal of Advanced Nursing* 18 (8): 1188–1192.

Atkins, S. and Schutz, S. (2013). Developing skills for reflective practice. In: *Reflective Practice in Nursing*, 5e (ed. C. Bulman and S. Schutz). Wiley-Blackwell.

Baillie, L. (ed.) (2014). *Developing Practical Nursing Skills*, 4e. CRC Press. Taylor & Francis Group. LLC.

Barchard, F. (2021). Exploring the role of reflection in nurse education and practice. *Nursing Standard* 37 (6).

Benner, P. (2001). *From Novice to Expert. Excellence and Power in Clinical Nursing Practice*, Commemorative Edition. New Jersey: Prentice Hall Health.

Bolton, G. and Delderfield, R. (2018). *Reflective Practice. Writing and Professional Development*, 5e. Sage.

Borton, (1970). *Reach, Touch and Teach*. London: Hutchinson.

Boud, D., Keogh, R., and Walker, D. (1985). *Reflection: Turning Experience into Learning*. London: Kogan Page.

Bridges J. and Wilkinson C. (2011). Achieving dignity for older people with dementia in hospital. *Nursing Standard* 25 (29): 42–47.

Brookfield, S.D. (2009). The concept of critical reflection: promises and contradictions. *European Journal of Social Work* 12: 293–304.

Brookfield, S.D. (2012). *Teaching for Critical Thinking*. Jossey-Bass. John Wiley & Sons.

Bulman, C. and Schutz, S. (2013). *Reflective Practice in Nursing*, 5e. Wiley–Blackwell.

Burnard, P. (1992). *Know Yourself! Self-Awareness Activities for Nurses*. Scutari Press. Royal College of Nursing.

Cambridge English Dictionary (2022). https://dictionary.cambridge.org/dictionary/english/assumption.

Cook, S.H. (2001). The self in self-awareness. *Learning Global Nursing Research* 29 (6): 1292–1299.

Csikszentmihalyi, M. (2002). *Flow. The Classic Work on How to Achieve Happiness*. Rider. The Random House Group Limited.

Dahlgren, M.A., Richardson, B., and Kalman, H. (2004). Redefining the reflective practitioner. In: *Developing Practice Knowledge for Health Professionals* (ed. J. Higgs, B. Richardson, and M.A. Dahlgren). Butterworth-Heinemann.

Danchev, A. (2016). (ed. and trans.) *The Letters of Paul Cezanne*, 253. Getty Publications. E-book: https://books.google.co.uk/books?id=gOprDQAAQBAJ&source=gbs_navlinks_s.

De Vries K. (2013). Communicating with older people with dementia. *Nursing Older People* 25 (4): 30–37.

Downs, M. and Bowers, B. (2008). *Excellence in Dementia Care. Research into Practice*, 223. Maidenhead: McGraw-Hill.

Driscoll, J. (1994). Reflective practice for practice – a framework of structured reflection for clinical areas. *Senior Nurse* 14 (1): 47–50.

Driscoll, J. (2007). *Practising Clinical Supervision: A Reflective Approach for Healthcare Professionals*. Edinburgh: Bailliere Tindall/Elsevier.

Duke, S. (2013). A personal exploration of reflective and clinical expertise. In: *Reflective Practice in Nursing*, 5e (ed. C. Bulman and S. Schutz). Wiley-Blackwell.

Eraut, M. (2007). Learning from other people in the workplace. *Oxford Review of Education* 33 (4): 403–422.

European Parkinson's Disease Association (2016). Caring and Parkinson's. https://www.epda.eu.com/living-well/caring-and-parkinsons/managing-movement-difficulties

Gibbs, G. (1988). *Learning by Doing: A Guide to Teaching and Learning Methods*. London: Further Education Unit.

Heron, M. and Corradini, E. (2020). A genre-based study of professional reflective writing in higher education. *Teaching in Higher Education*. https://doi.org/10.1080/13562517.2020.1824178.

Higgs, J. and Titchen, A. (2001). *Professional Practice in Health, Education and the Creative Arts*. Blackwell Science.

Howatson-Jones, L. (2016). *Reflective Practice in Nursing*, 3e. Sage. Learning Matters.

Jack, K. and Smith, A. (2007). Promoting self-awareness in nurses to improve nursing practice. *Nursing Standard* 21 (32): 47–52.

Jarvis, P. (2006). *Towards a Comprehensive Theory of Human Learning: Lifelong Learning and the Learning Society*, 1. London: Routledge.

Jarvis, P. (2010). *Adult Education and Lifelong Learning: Theory and Practice*. London: Routledge.

Jasper, M. (2013). *Beginning Reflective Practice*. UK: Cengage Learning.

Johns, C. (2009). *Becoming a Reflective Practitioner*. Wiley–Blackwell.

Kolb, D.A. (1984). *Experiential Learning - Experience as the Source of Learning and Development*. New Jersey: Prentice Hall.

Lister, S., Hofland, J., and Grafton, H. (eds.) (2020). *The Royal Marsden Manual of Clinical Nursing Procedures*, 10e. Wiley Blackwell.

Luft, J. and Ingham, H. (1955). *The Johari Window, a Graphic Model of Interpersonal Awareness*.

Mann, K., Gordon, J., and MacLeod, A. (2009). Reflection and reflective practice in health professions education: a systematic review. *Advances in Health Science Education* 14: 595–621.

McNamara, G. (2016). Communicating to patients with Alzheimer's. *Nursing in Practice*. https://www.nursinginpractice.com/clinical/addiction-and-mental-health/mental-health/communicating-to-patients-with-alzheimers.

Mezirow, J. (2000). *Learning as Transformation: Critical Perspectives on a Theory in Progress*. San Francisco: Jossey Bass.

Moon, J. and Fowler, J. (2008). There is a story to be told: a framework for the conception for story in higher education and professional development. *Nurse Education Today* 28: 232e239.

National Institute for Health and Care Excellence (2017). Parkinson's disease in adults: NICE guideline NG71. https://www.nice.org.uk/guidance/ng71/evidence/full-guideline-pdf-4538466253.

National Health Service (2020). Communicating with someone with dementia. *Dementia Guide* http://www.nhs.uk.

NHS (2021). Professional nurse advocate A-EQUIP model. *A model of clinical supervision for nurses*. www.england.nhs.uk/publication/professional-nurse-advocate-a-equip-model-a-model-of-clinical-supervision-for-nurses.

Nightingale, F. (1860). *Notes on Nursing*. D. Appleton and Company.

Nightingale, F. (1969). *Notes on Nursing*. Dover Publications. (Republication from Nightingale F (1860). Notes on Nursing. D. Appleton and Company.)

Nursing and Midwifery Council (2016). *Revalidation*. NMC.

Nursing and Midwifery Council (2018). *Future Nurse: Standards of Proficiency for Registered Nurses*. NMC.

O'Sullivan, E., O'Neill, E., and Hathaway, M. (2016). *Transformative Learning: Fostering Educational Vision in the 21st Century*, 2e. Zed books.

Oelofsen, N. (2012). *Developing Reflective Practice. A Guide for Students and Practitioners of Health and Social Care*. Banbury: Lantern Publishing Limited.

Rasheed, S.P. (2015). Self-Awareness as a Therapeutic Tool for Nurse/Client Relationship. *International Journal of Caring Science* 8 (1): 211.

Rolfe, G., Freshwater, D., and Jasper, M. (2001). *Critical Reflection for Nursing and the Helping Professions.: A User's Guide*. Basingstoke: Palgrave.

Rolfe, G., Jasper, M., and Freshwater, D. (2011). *Critical Reflection in Practice: Generating Knowledge for Care*, 2e. Palgrave Macmillan.

Schon, D.A. (1987). *Educating the Reflective Practitioner*. San Francisco: Jossey-Bass.

Schon, D.A. (1991). *The Reflective Practitioner. How Professionals Think in Action*. Arena. Ashgate Publishing Limited.

Schutz, S. (2013). Assessing and evaluating reflection. In: *Reflective Practice in Nursing*, 5e (ed. C. Bulman and S. Schutz). Wiley-Blackwell.

Scriven, A. (2017). *Ewles & Simnett's Promoting Health Practical Guide*, 7e. Edinburgh: Elsevier.

Storr, W. (2019). *The Science of Storytelling: Why Stories Make Us Human, and How to Tell Them Better*. London: Collins.

Tate, S. (2013). Writing to learn; writing reflectively. In: *Reflective Practice in Nursing*, 5e (ed. C. Bulman and S. Schutz). Wiley-Blackwell.

Williams S. and Herman R. (2011) Linking resident behaviour to dementia care communication: effects of emotional tone. *Behaviour Therapy* 42 (1): 42–46.

Williams, K.N., Herman, R., Gajewski, B., and Wilson, K. (2009). Elderspeak communication: impact on dementia care. *American Journal of Alzheimer's Disease* 24 (1): 11–20.

CHAPTER 6

Caring for Yourself

Our training teaches us that nursing is a profession where you must put others before yourself. This becomes ingrained as a code of practice or learnt behaviour. It is this that enables us to engage in the emotional labour of nursing, giving of our time, energy and skills unconditionally and in response to the needs of those in our care. Such altruism brings its own rewards and personal fulfilment, of course, but it also comes at a cost. Whether you have little or no post-registration experience or whether you have many nursing years behind you, you will know the strain that nursing work can bring. Perhaps you left because you felt that you could give no more. A NMC survey in 2019–2020 indicated that of the 21,800 nurses who left the register during this timeframe, one in five nurses cited poor mental health and stress as their reason for leaving (NMC 2020). In Chapter 3 we discussed the importance of knowing yourself and understanding your own needs and aims in the context of returning to practice. This chapter takes those insights forward. Reflecting on why you left the profession will help you to take care of yourself when you re-enter the nursing workforce.

Vacancies within the NHS remain at a high level with almost 39,000 nursing posts recorded as unfilled in June 2021 (NHS Digital 2022). Many nurses are concerned about working conditions and morale. Indications from the Building a Better Future survey (RCN 2020) show the following as major factors:

- higher pay (73% of staff)
- improved staffing levels (50%)
- safe working conditions (45%)
- adequate equipment and materials (43%)

Returning to Nursing Practice: Confidence and Competence, First Edition. Ros Wray and Mary Kitson.
© 2023 John Wiley & Sons Ltd. Published 2023 by John Wiley & Sons Ltd.

Nursing is a demanding profession. There are high expectations from ourselves, employers and patients, yet we are often undervalued in monetary terms. Many nurses have felt pressured by this challenge and leave to rethink their careers (Coates and Macfadyen 2021). The recent pandemic exposed the reality of these issues. Kinnair (2020) has suggested that the clapping is now over, and it is time the government heard the voices of UK nurses and worked to ensure that nursing is supported, valued and viewed as an attractive career option.

The NHS Constitution (2021) reinforces the core values of the founding scheme in 1948 which saw the NHS as a comprehensive service, freely available to all and access based on clinical need rather than ability to pay. Along with a raised awareness of patient safety and the necessary investment required to ensure sustainability in healthcare provision for the ever-changing complex needs of the population, there is also an increasing focus on and recognition of the people delivering this care. Consequently, this may be an exciting time to consider returning to your chosen career. 'Respect, dignity, compassion and care should be at the core of how patients and staff are treated not only because that is the right thing to do but because patient safety, experience and outcomes are all improved when staff are valued, empowered and supported' (The NHS Constitution 2021).

Over a quarter of nurses decide to take a career break due to personal circumstances (NMC 2020), and often individual factors spur their return. Children may be less dependent, a breakdown in relationships may necessitate reconsideration of financial income, or a change in carer responsibilities may bring more freedom. Whatever the reasons for leaving and returning, some pressures and concerns will still exist. However, forewarned is forearmed. Passion for nursing still prevails (Cope et al. 2016) and you are returning to nursing with the added self-insight that comes with maturity. It is likely that you will already have a range of tried and tested strategies that help you to care for yourself. Here, we hope to add to this collection, offering tips and ideas to help combat any stressors felt during your return journey.

COURSE PROGRESSION POINTS

Return to Practice courses are challenging. You will feel stretched on all fronts – physically, mentally and emotionally. Consequently, it will also test those closest to you. Partners, children, friends and parents may all be affected. Communication is vital, so that all can understand how best to be supportive.

Each course has an individual shape and momentum. If yours starts with a bulk of induction study days (and most do), you may feel overloaded with information, and tired from travelling unfamiliar routes to university campuses. The first day back in a clinical setting may bring a twist of anxiety but also a feeling of relief and achievement. As course tutors we have observed that most students seem more relaxed after a few weeks in placement. However, that is not to deny that your first days in practice may feel uncomfortable and disorientating as you come to grips with a faster pace of care delivery and perceive changes in nursing culture. As highlighted earlier, planning and preparation will help you through. Many courses are structured to encourage students to share their first impressions of practice with each other. Course educators and practice teams understand the importance of peer support and will work to create opportunities for returners to come together to listen to each other's placement experiences. This sharing of stories helps to establish camaraderie and a sense of belonging (Bolton and Delderfield 2018).

Words of Wisdom

I think another area that helped myself was that the group on the course agreed to set up a chat via message, which meant we could all gain from each other top tips or things that did not work for us. I will be forever grateful for meeting this wonderful group of people, all having similar worries, doubts and finally achievements too.

Course midpoints can mark a crucial time. At this juncture there can be a blind foggy feeling – you are no longer new, but the endpoint is still out of sight. Support from fellow students is always welcome; however, comparisons with the progress of others can be unhelpful, and can even lead to disillusionment and self-doubt. It is important to remember that you are following your own personal journey. Inevitably, some returners will find themselves tested more than others. Practice environments can suddenly dip into a difficult period perhaps due to staff sickness or heavy workloads. Personal factors, such as ill health or unforeseen family events, can present added challenges. Others may find that things flow along with ease. This is just the way it is, and each will find their way provided help is sought as needed. Course and practice teams are very supportive, but need to be aware of potential problems, so do communicate with them if you have concerns.

Midway through, students are fully engaged in practice and academic work and can start to feel overwhelmed by the pressure of juggling both simultaneously. Concerns about meeting practice requirements and a tendency to over-think academic assignments can add to the stress. A timely and reassuring chat with a course tutor can help to keep things in proportion, and midpoint assessment in practice will provide concrete feedback on achievement so far with clear directions on what to focus on next. As you will perhaps remember from previous mentoring roles, feedback should be timely, balanced and objective. There may be some aspects that you will need to improve; however, constructive criticism should be sandwiched between positives. It is true, of course, that some assessors and supervisors may be more adept at delivering these kinds of comments than others. It is important not let negative feedback push you off track. Be open and receptive and have a dialogue about what has been said as this may help to give you focus and direction. Nonetheless, there will be moments of hesitation and doubt.

> **Words of Wisdom**
>
> Sometimes I would have a challenging shift, either I felt I had not helped a patient as much as I wanted to or that my knowledge was lacking. I tried to remind myself that my mentor knew I was a return to practice student even though in my head I felt I should be fully qualified! I went away and researched and began the next shift armed with new knowledge which I could often implement immediately.

Here is the same student towards completion of placement!

> **Words of Wisdom**
>
> After I found my feet, I realised that I had knowledge I could share. By the time I left, some of the community support workers and younger staff nurses were asking me for support!

Placement may be exhausting physically, mentally and emotionally, but pacing yourself and staying organised will help to keep everything in perspective. Many students take a few days break halfway through – this can make all the difference.

Course endpoints bring assignment deadlines and naturally this can be stressful. There is no shame in the realisation that academic writing may not be one of your strengths. One of our returners exclaimed to the rest of her group that the most academic thing she had written in the last ten years was a shopping list! This made us all laugh, breaking the ice, and giving other students the confidence to voice their own anxieties. Some students plan to complete their work early, saving themselves the pressures of a last-minute rush. This may not be possible for everyone despite best laid plans! However, forward planning of some kind and good organisation are helpful. Try not to feel intimidated by the volume of work that you have taken on; as we have said many times, it is essential to let tutors and placement staff know if circumstances start to hinder your progress.

SELF-CARE: MANAGING YOUR WELL-BEING

The stress of modern living can be relentless as the recent COVID-19 pandemic has highlighted and therefore the ability to maintain well-being has become something of an art. This art comes with an increasing set of recommended skills and a new language: resilience, mindfulness, sleep hygiene, 'being brilliant' and keeping safe – to name a few. There is much here of value, and this chapter will explore some useful strategies. However, we advise a measured response, selecting only what feels right for you. Opening too many doors into this world can bring its own kind of pressure and self-expectation.

As you prepare for your return to nursing, consider also how you can best care for yourself by weighing personal strengths and potential challenges. Self-care and self-compassion are fundamental to how we are engaging with those around us both on a personal and professional level (RCN 2021a). Our nursing code reminds us to look to our own health as well of those of others (NMC 2018a). The notion of self-care is fundamental to good practice. Before we can care for others safely and effectively, we must be able to care for ourselves. This is not new to the caring professions; in counselling, for example, practitioners understand the need to look to their personal well-being.

The RCN 'Healthy workplace, healthy you' assessment is a helpful resource which encourages a holistic approach to self-care (RCN 2021a). You are asked to rate a series of statements based on your body, mind, heart, spirit, work, career and, most fundamentally, balance. Apart from career (addressed in Chapter 8), we have structured this chapter broadly around these areas.

BODY: PHYSICAL WELL-BEING

Nursing is hard work. Many returning nurses remark on how tired they feel after their first days back in practice. You will remember the physical toll of long shifts, but your bodies may not have experienced this kind of challenge for some years. As one recent returner commented, 'It takes a while to recover that muscle memory.' Whilst some students may feel compelled to get ahead, rushing at the start can be counterproductive and result in unnecessary pressure. We would advise that you take your time as you reacclimatise, balancing the demands of practice placements with rest and sleep.

Most of us require seven or eight hours of sleep to function well. However, studies show that nurses tend to sleep less than the rest of the population (Eanes 2015). Irregular shift patterns and the emotional intensity of nursing work can lead to chronic sleep deprivation; this, in turn, leads to mounting fatigue and a lack of concentration which can increase the incidence of workplace errors and have an impact on patient safety (Caruso et al. 2019; Sun et al. 2020). These studies highlight strong links between poor physical health, insomnia, compassion fatigue and burnout. Rest, therefore, is crucial. This is not just about a good night's sleep, but also includes restorative breaks during a working shift. The COVID-19 lockdowns have underlined our mutual need for social interaction with colleagues and friends. When staff get caught up in a cycle of busyness, missed meal breaks can become the norm exacting a negative effect on our own well-being and on patient health outcomes (Witkoski and Dickson 2010). Sometimes a cultural shift is required for staff to rethink and decide to physically remove themselves from the area for a brief interval. However, if your break becomes overdue, a well-timed and thoughtful reminder is welcomed. It is your right to take regular breaks in placement so do not soldier on uncomfortably.

Remember the basics of good nutrition and hydration. Increased physical activity requires fuel. Try to maintain good dietary habits, making time for proper food and mealtimes with loved ones. This may sound obvious, but it is easy to slip into convenience eating and short-cut snacking when busy. If meal breaks at work are forfeited, quick fixes are tempting in the form of sugary snacks and drinks. A recent article in the Nursing Standard pointed to increasing concerns about overweight issues in the nursing profession; one in four nurses has a BMI of over 30, and this, as we know, sets a precedence for long-term health implications (Trueland 2022). As nurses we also understand the role of hydration in sustaining health. However, research shows that even mild dehydration in healthy adults and children is very common (Gandy 2012). Not drinking sufficiently can affect cognitive ability, lower our mood and cause fatigue (Adan 2012; Masento et al. 2014). As we advocate for patients, explaining the importance of daily exercise, being well-hydrated and eating a varied diet, we must also take note and not forget our own health!

Here are a few practical tips:

- Plan your lunch the night before. Take with you packed food and keep this varied. Soups, sandwiches, salads and even leftovers from the day before can all be easy options.
- Take your breaks.
- Remember that a protein-rich breakfast will help sustain energy levels.
- Walk for twenty minutes every day.
- Snack on fruit.
- Keep hydrated.

Words of Wisdom

Plan dedicated, regular, protected time to complete the course requirements to help you meet deadlines. To do this, consider who can help you at home to free up the mental capacity and new commitments on your time that you will need as you adjust to returning to learning mode. Can anyone else relieve you of existing non- work time responsibilities for the duration of the course? Ask for what you need and be specific. Enjoy being free of the responsibilities of washing, cooking and cleaning for a while- it's great! I asked my husband to help more with household jobs that were normally my responsibility. I didn't necessarily let him know when I was having a less pressurised week!

MIND: MENTAL WELL-BEING

In the past, musculoskeletal conditions have tended to be at the root of most health-related problems for nurses. As Hulatt (2019) reports, there was a time when back problems were seen as an occupational hazard of the role; now however, stress and poor mental well-being are moving to the forefront of issues for health service workers.

Our mental health is ever-fluctuating, sensitive and responsive as we pass through various encounters and stages in our lives. However, despite much discussion, there is no consensus on a clear definition (Galderisi et al. 2015). Most recently, the World Health Organisation described a state of mental well-being as one which 'enables people to cope with stresses of life, realise their abilities, learn well and work well and contribute to their community' (WHO 2022). All agree that our mental health plays a major role in our general well-being and sense of happiness, so it is important to be aware of it and to appreciate that some days we will feel we can climb mountains and on others we will feel like we are holding on by our fingertips. Nurses are responsible for the health and well-being of other people so to function effectively we must try to maintain our own mental well-being (Tennant et al. 2007; Xie et al. 2011).

One initiative is Mental Health First Aid training. These courses were originally established in Australia in 2000 by married couple, Betty Kitchner and Anthony Jorm, both of whom have backgrounds in health education and mental health literacy (Kitchener and Jorm 2008). The training has since been adopted internationally to educate people to recognise and support those suffering with deteriorating mental health. The principle is based on the concept of physical first aid where prompt recognition of a problem facilitates a quick response. The stigma that surrounds mental health can prevent people from seeking timely intervention. Evidence indicates that this MHFA initiative is effective in raising awareness and knowledge, instilling people with the confidence to start conversations with family members or colleagues in mental health crisis situations (MHFA 2019). We have recently introduced the two-day MHFA course for returning nurses who found it insightful. Ultimately it proved to be highly significant to their practice experience where they felt better able to understand and support those in their care.

Universities can provide a range of additional support services for those who suffer with mental health conditions. Teams of counsellors and mental health advisers are trained and experienced to understand the stress points in student life and how these can challenge mental health well-being. Support is focused on what will relieve pressure so that students are able to stay on courses and achieve success. Whilst Return to Practice courses are short and usually part time, and mature learners may already have well-established support networks and insight into existing mental health issues, it is worth noting that this help is readily available. The demands of returning to nursing can exact an unexpected toll, pushing some towards unrealistic self-expectation or perfectionism. For others it may be that personal circumstances suddenly make course attendance difficult. If you find yourself struggling with low mood or a sense of panic, it is important to share this with your course team or personal tutor. There is a repertoire of measures that can be used to give space for recovery, whether this amounts to a few weeks of time-out or a longer study break. Many of our students have done just this, going on to complete the course successfully when their lives return to a more manageable norm.

Mindfulness

Mindfulness is the opposite of automatic pilot. It connects you to the here and now, offering the potential to reduce stress and increase positive emotions. Whilst some suggest that simple breathing exercises help to prepare for the experience, there is no magic switch to flip a racing mind to one that is calm and serene and allows us to lay down tools and relax. Like all new skills it takes a little practice.

At the core of mindfulness is the concept of being present and receptive to what is happening in the moment. Instead of rushing through the task with our minds elsewhere, taking the time to focus on simple activities like washing up can bring calm. We start to really appreciate the feel of the soapy water and the smell of the washing up liquid. Breathing deeply whilst you are doing this – inhaling and exhaling – slows us down, allowing any thoughts or feelings to come to the fore, and then disperse. It is a kind of informal meditation which can be undertaken anywhere. Just simply pausing to notice our surroundings can help us to refocus, benefitting our well-being and thereby those around us. The following simple exercise provides a taster (literally!) and may surprise those who have not tried mindfulness before. If raisins are not your thing, please do find something more to your liking.

Raisin Mindfulness Exercise

Find a quiet spot where you can sit and relax. Once you are comfortable, pick up the raisin and hold it in your hand.

- **LOOK at the raisin.** Really concentrate and focus on it; pick out all the details – the colour, areas of light and shade, any ridges or shine.
- **TOUCH the raisin.** Feel its smallness in your palm. Explore the texture with your fingers.
- **SMELL the raisin.** Bring it close to your nose and breathe deeply in and out, inhaling the smell of the raisin.
- **TASTE the raisin.** Turn it over in your mouth and feel its texture on the roof of your mouth. Gently bite into it, without swallowing it yet. Concentrate on the sensations just released into your mouth. How does it taste? How does this develop as the moments pass? How has the raisin changed? Do the smaller pieces of fruit feel different?
- **HEAR the sounds** you make as you chew it and swallow. Focus on the sensation of the raisin going into your tummy. Now take a moment to notice how your whole body feels. Slowly start to awaken your mind. Gently move the hands and feet a little, slowly open your eyes and breathe deeply. https://www.youtube.com/watch?v=1umGZ8S8tHo

---

Studies suggest that mindfulness practised by people in various professional roles can help to manage work-related stress (Foureur et al. 2013; Burton et al. 2016). The approach has also been linked to the strengthening of resilience attributes and reduction in the incidence of burnout (Turner 2009; Bolton 2010). However, Barratt and Wagstaffe (2018) caution that in conjunction with the positive benefits experienced, it is possible that troubling thoughts and experiences may also surface and be difficult to manage. If this is the case, they suggest that input from a more experienced practitioner may be advisable. It is important to choose what works best for you. Here are some thoughts from one of our returning students:

Words of Wisdom

Mindfulness training has allowed me to develop my self-awareness and gain the ability to take a step back and assess a situation. It can be used for self-care and is something I find extremely useful in my day-to-day life as it allows me to focus on the present.

Mindfulness can enhance our connections with patients. It sits with active listening and therapeutic presence, helping us to still the internal chatter and endless dashing and racing to the next task. Patients feel cared for if we can be with them, hearing what is being said and not said, rather than churning over the lists of things we need to do. Being mindful can also mean that we become present with or aware of our own emotions, not to then suppress any negative feelings, but to learn to deal with them more adeptly. In the extract below, one returner describes a troubling conversation from early in her practice placement. Keen to provide supportive answers for an oncology patient who has queries about her forthcoming chemotherapy treatment, the student struggles to respond fully, hampered by a sense of the limitations of her role.

Returner's Reflection

I did not contribute much to the conversation and did not ask many questions. This made me feel uncomfortable. My thoughts were more focused on what I was going to say to Mrs. A rather than what she was saying. Mrs. A may perhaps have just required a sympathetic ear; and it is important for me to acknowledge that although I felt inadequate in this situation and had negative feelings, Mrs. A may well have benefitted from just being able to talk. However, I was too caught up in my own anxieties to consider these things at the time. Internal distractions became a barrier to effective listening.

Flow

First impressions may see flow as almost the reverse of mindfulness. It suggests such a full immersion in an activity that we lose a sense of the present. We talk of burying ourselves in a book only to emerge two hours later in utter surprise that so much time has passed! Long walks or listening to a favourite piece of music can be sensed in a similar way. Time feels altered because we are so involved in what we are doing. There is no room for everyday worries or self-consciousness. Csikszentmihalyi's extensive research leads him to conclude that 'being able to forget temporarily who we are seems to be very enjoyable' (2002, p. 64). His flow theory points to the fact that certain experiences have the power to absorb us completely, and that this can feel exhilarating.

Like mindfulness (arguably, a part of 'flow') this profound focus on something other than self is not reserved for extreme or outlandish activities. We are talking here of simple hobbies and sports such as gardening, yoga, knitting, swimming, running, crafts, cooking, dancing, colouring pictures or playing chess. The key message is that any kind of activity or pursuit that brings you 'flow' will also bring happiness and a sense of well-being, helping to balance the pressures of daily life, work and study.

Words of Wisdom

Allow yourself some time for you, whatever that may be – a hobby or interest. I am certain mine of running helped me to keep going, although finding the time was more challenging. This will be a good activity to continue with in the nursing workforce.

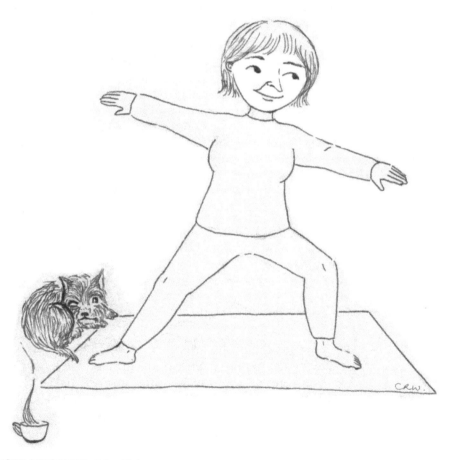

ILLUSTRATION NO. 6.1   Doing yoga.

Relaxation Therapies

Non-conventional therapies can range from established alternative treatments such as acupuncture and homeopathy to more complementary approaches which include massage, meditation and aromatherapy. Whilst quantitative science may still question the validity of some of these therapies, members of the public often find them beneficial.

An in-depth discussion of the many therapies on offer is beyond the scope of this book. Instead, our focus is on encouraging whatever you find most relaxing whether it be listening to music, or a good soak in a hot bath. Remembering and prioritising the things that we know do us good is not always easy, especially when we are busy. Course days will feel long, other tasks will intrude, demanding attention, and suddenly the moment has gone. Here, therefore, are two quick and simple well-being exercises that can be undertaken almost anywhere and may help to retrieve a little calm.

We connect with the world through our five senses, and these provide the access points for many therapeutic approaches. First and foremost, however, comes breathing. It is the key to life and the foundation for most relaxation therapies. The following exercise demonstrates diaphragmatic breathing, a technique which helps to combat stress by reducing cortisol levels (Ma et al. 2017).

Breathing Exercise

Find a comfortable position. Most people find either sitting or lying down works best.

Place the palm of both hands on your tummy.

Close your eyes and take a few seconds to centre yourself.

Focus on your breath.

As you breathe in, let your tummy rise beneath your hands. Hold this for a few comfortable moments. Then as you breathe out, let your tummy fall.

Repeat this movement when the next breath comes, letting your tummy rise, and then fall, as you inhale and exhale.

Continue the exercise for several minutes and then finish, slowly opening your eyes.

For most people, this method slows and deepens breathing, easing both body and mind. The diaphragm fully contracts and relaxes, and the base of the lungs expand, mimicking how we tend to breathe during sleep. Diaphragmatic breathing requires less effort than chest breathing (Ma et al. 2017). Being aware of the number of breaths in a minute before and during the exercise will demonstrate its efficacy. However, it does not work for everyone. Some find it difficult to focus on their breath and may therefore find the next exercise more helpful. Visualisation techniques work to settle the mind by enhancing awareness and focus. They are sometimes used in meditation.

Visualisation

Find a comfortable position, either sitting or lying down. Make sure that your hands, arms, legs and feet feel supported. Check that your neck and shoulders are in a relaxed position.

Close your eyes and become aware of your breathing. Take a few moments to centre yourself by breathing slowly and deeply.

Imagine that you are a rosebush.... What colour are the roses? ...Do they have a fragrance? .... Are there many layers of petals or just a few? Can you see the centre of the roses? ... What do your stems and leaves look like? ... Where are you growing? ... Imagine your roots? How do they feel in the soil?

What is it like being a rosebush? ... How does it feel when it rains?

Follow your imagination where it takes you...

When you are ready to stop, let the image go. Become aware again of your body. In your own time, open your eyes.

Pietroni (1986)

SPIRITUAL WELL-BEING

In nursing, we are counselled to treat our patients holistically, taking account of their physical, psychological, social and spiritual needs (NMC 2018a). Of course, spiritual well-being means different things to different people and is not necessarily synonymous with religious faith. For many, though, spirituality is diverse and complex, connecting to deep-rooted values. Nursing models have sought to embrace the concept of spirituality, reminding us of its importance and aligning it with the recovery of health (Roy 1980; Roper et al. 1980). However, such is the diversity of belief systems that as nurses we can find it difficult to meet the needs of our patients. Research by Funning (2010) highlighted nurses felt ill prepared to manage patients' spiritual needs but they believed spiritual care was aligned to the core values of nursing practice: respect, dignity and compassion. This provides guidance, echoing the core nursing value of person-centred care.

Nurses may have challenges reconciling their own beliefs with the opposing views and opinions of others at vulnerable times. A safe passage through may lie in empathising and acknowledging strength of feelings, rather than trying to offer solutions and explanations. These are attributes which we also need to apply to our own everyday lives. Recognising what is important to us may help us to find anchor on difficult days. A quiet ten minutes listening to the birds or the leaves in the trees can settle our own spirits.

HEART: EMOTIONAL WELL-BEING

Due to the nature of caring nursing has been identified as being underpinned by emotional labour. This phrase was initially coined in 1983 by American sociologist, Arlie Hochschild, in her book *The Managed Heart*. Occupations which require emotional labour are made up of three components: intensive contact with the public, invoking emotional states in others, and the existence of rules or codes that guide how we behave (Hochschild 1983). The initial expression was related to the service industries, especially airline cabin staff where there was an organisational expectation that personnel provide a smiling 'customer is right' attitude.

The emotional labour of nursing is well documented (Hochschild 1983; Smith 1992; Smith and Gray 2001; Dewar and Christley 2013). Regardless of the context, our everyday work involves interacting with patients and families, helping them to face challenging, and sometimes, life-changing situations. We focus on supporting them, often prioritising their needs above our own. This responsibility can be extremely stressful and self-protection strategies can manifest. Patients rate interpersonal relationships higher than clinical competence and technical skills (Wysong and Driver 2009; RCN 2010). However, when feelings of frustration, anger, grief or even fear become overwhelming, nurses tend to cope by dividing labour into tasks to minimise nurse–patient interaction (Menzies 1960 cited in Smith 2012). We all have memories of emotionally stressful days in practice and perhaps the sense at the time that no one prepared us for this role.

Recent acknowledgement has come in NHS The People Plan (2020), a publication triggered by the experiences of NHS workers paid and voluntary across the sector during the COVID-19 pandemic. This document pays tribute to those who work in healthcare, urging an ethos of compassion and belonging. It goes further to set out an NHS People Promise which aims to secure confidence in expressing a voice about fair and flexible working, feeling healthy and safe and being deserving of thanks (NHS England 2020). This is the well-intentioned, emotive language of an employer to its workers during a time of acute stress and trauma. Yet, it also underscores the need to ensure, by continuous review, that healthcare environments for employees and students remain positive and conducive to caring and learning. At the heart of this endeavour lies each individual and the need we all have to take care of each other.

Gratitude and appreciation are generally conveyed by saying 'Thank you'. These small words have a powerful impact. It is well established that the expression of gratitude is related to physical and mental well-being (Henning et al. 2017) and therefore something that we need to incorporate into our daily lives. Collaborative teamwork operates both ways in effecting a sense of individual well-being. Practice Assessors and Supervisors also need to receive positive feedback so any messages of thanks that you can give them will mean a great deal. In their study Coates and MacFadyen (2021) noted that peer support from returners to the profession is especially valued by clinical staff. Cheng et al. (2015) reported a 28% reduction in perceived stress and 16% reduction in depression when they implemented a gratitude intervention amongst healthcare workers.

The emotions of appreciation and gratitude have a positive impact on the brain, altering neural structures to make us feel happier and more resilient (Fox et al. 2015). In one fascinating study, ECG recordings show that the heart and brain are interlinked or tuned to each other (McCraty and Childre 2004). Our internal physiological rhythms function at their best when we are happy. The more we initiate appreciative responses the more these patterns establish, enabling us to withstand the impact of daily irritations and frustrations. The challenge is to consciously choose a positive attitude. McCraty and Childre (2004) explain that patterns of behaviour can just as easily fix into habitual cynicism or low morale which can be draining for the person concerned and those around them. The motivational training and resources generated by the Art of Being Brilliant campaign promote positive psychology through the sharing of simple, logical life-improving suggestions (Cope 2017). This strategy has seven key areas that underpin the initiative – Why be ordinary when you can be brilliant? They provide a guide for positive thinking and are as follows:

- Choosing to be positive
- Taking personal responsibility
- Going the extra mile
- Bouncebackability (resilience)
- Understanding you impact (emotional intelligence)
- Appreciation and gratitude
- Celebration of achievement

Work

So much of how we perform in our roles is impacted by our workplace. It is important that the environment and organisational ethos is healthy and facilitates staff well-being. You may not have the opportunity to be too specific or selective in securing a placement to undertake your supervised practice as placements are facilitated with universities and aligned Trusts. However, all placements are audited for their suitability as an educational environment which can support students to achieve programme learning outcomes, and efforts are made to match with your previous experience or current circumstances. Your practice placement will be short in duration, but potentially could lead to an offer of employment on completion. Before jumping in, ask yourself a few questions. Is this a healthy setting for me to work in? How is staff morale? What are the retention rates? If the answers are not favourable, there may be alternative options.

The Code (2018) clearly identifies the organisational and professional responsibilities required to ensure systems are in place to support a healthy working environment in which staff can thrive. The RCN defines a healthy workplace as 'one which offers fair pay and rewards and has high quality employment practices and procedures which

- are inclusive,
- promote a good work-life balance,
- protect and promote employees' physical and psychological health,

- design jobs which provide employees with autonomy and control,
- provide equitable access to training and learning and development.'

(RCN Healthy Workplace Toolkit RCN 2021a, p. 4)

Reporting Practice Concerns

Nurses have a moral and ethical duty to speak up about any issues of concern. Sadly, mistakes can happen due to various factors such as lack of knowledge, inadequate resources, poor communication or negligence. As returning nurses, you will know that we have a duty of care to our patients, ensuring that we practise safely and effectively to promote their well-being.

When errors occur, it is crucial that they are reported and recorded. We must be open and transparent whether the incident relates to our own practice or those of others. This is a stressful area for all of us. However, Francis (2015) highlighted that having the courage to voice concerns is crucial to patient safety and quality of care. There are various channels of communication and university systems in place to support you in this process primarily underpinned by our duty of candour, formalised within the NMC Code since 2015. Written guidance on the process of managing concerns was updated in 2022, and comes in two parts:

1. *Nurses, midwives and nursing associates have a duty to be open and honest with the people who use services, and those close to them. This includes explaining when and why things have gone wrong and apologising to them.*
2. *Professionals also have a duty to report incidents, and be open and honest with their colleagues, managers, and employers. This might include their health board, trust or head office, and the NMC.*

(NMC 2022)

RESILIENCE

Resilience is a word that has recently become very popular throughout society and within organisations. The original term was linked to work undertaken by child psychologists whose research in the 70s and 80s raised questions about why some children were able to surmount adverse circumstances, and others were not. A dictionary definition portrays resilience as the capacity to recover quickly from difficulties or describes the ability of a material 'to resume its original shape or position after being bent, stretched, or compressed' (*The Free Dictionary*, n.d.).

The concept is a familiar one. How often have we cajoled children after a fall – 'Oops! You will be fine' or 'Think of the positives; things could be worse' or even, 'Tomorrow is another day'. Many of us have grown up with these expressions ingrained, setting up expectations that we must keep strong and bounce back. Whilst the term 'resilience' is used widely across a range of disciplines and workplaces, its meaning in these contexts remains complicated and ambivalent (Aburn et al. 2016). In relation to nursing, Hart et al. (2014) suggest that resilience is linked to professional challenges that nurses encounter in their daily work. It tends to be viewed as the individual's ability to cope and keep on coping. Nurses are expected to recognise the need to enhance their personal resilience. The NMC Future Nurse standards (2018b) require the 21st century nurse to be an emotionally intelligent and resilient individual. However, as we have already discussed, resource pressures and the pace of change in healthcare can present serious challenges, with patients becoming even more vulnerable in settings that feel stressful and chaotic (Martin 2018, p. 152). Aburn et al. (2016) identify that both patients and carers struggle to sustain resilience in times of crisis, and others go further, criticising the use of the buzzword 'resilience' because it implies that failure to cope is due to a lack of personal attributes rather than resulting from wider factors such as systemic and organisational shortfalls (Dall'Ora 2020).

Research indicates that personal understanding of the concept of resilience is diverse with each of us interpreting it in different ways (Grant et al. 2013). It is generally felt not be an inherent aspect of character, but something akin to a skill that we can develop and strengthen (Beddoe et al. 2013). Personal resilience grows as we come to know ourselves and understand where our challenges lie and what helps us to feel strong. Importantly, it is seen as dynamic, fluid and changing from hour to hour (Aburn et al. 2016; Henshall et al. 2020). There may be days when we will feel more able to cope, and other times when we must step back and ask for support. Resilience should not be about working harder. Saying 'no' sometimes is crucial to well-being (Trueland 2017).

Within organisations the focus is beginning to lean towards supporting nurses to raise concerns and be assertive about poor work environments. Although you may not realise it, you may have some of the skills required to help this shift. Your experience, maturity and life skills are likely to push you to advocate for yourself and others in clinical settings, even though this may sound daunting. The current climate with its staffing and resource issues requires us to be assertive in seeking the necessary support to do our jobs well. This is not to expect you to bring about major change, but just to remind you of the strengths you have now compared with how you may have felt on leaving the clinical setting some years ago. McDonald et al. (2016) propose that resilience helps us to maintain and sustain a fulfilling career. They stress the significance of the competencies and factors that underpin resilience such as reflective learning, self-awareness and supportive structures such as clinical supervision.

Words of Wisdom

The placement progressed, and I grew in confidence as my skills improved. Interestingly, I noticed that the combination of the life skills I had acquired during my time away from nursing plus my renewed clinical expertise gave me a resilience I had not had before. Managing challenging situations did not seem as challenging as they once had.

Some returners may not have an inbuilt support network. They may be single parents who have decided to return to a career which offers solid financial stability. The journey's end may bring solutions, but the travelling may be arduous. In these situations, it is vital to ask for help. Once you seek support, responses can come from unexpected quarters. Remember, too, that in educational environments supportive mechanisms are in place from tutors and peers. Relationships soon develop as students seek to acquire and share knowledge and skills together (Burton et al. 2011). We have written much about peer support and its value in reducing stress for returning nurses. Lasting friendships are often forged within weeks.

Words of Wisdom

We had a cohort social media group which proved invaluable. We were in contact with each other once the in-person sessions had finished and continued to swap tips and ideas as we finished our writing. If you think you are the only one who is struggling, you can bet someone else is too!

On a more formal level, there have been positive moves to embed well-being strategies into the nurse education curriculum. Resilience is explained as an approach to self-care that can moderate stress and be beneficial to nursing students and those in their care (Davies 2020). Ultimately, one of the reasons it is crucial to cultivate resilience and assertiveness in healthcare professionals is to combat the impact and consequences of burn out and compassion fatigue. These emotional states are clearly exacerbated by nurses feeling responsible for workplace failures and this will be discussed later in the chapter.

Wobble Rooms

In response to the recent strain and emotional impact of the COVID-19 pandemic, attempts have been made to implement support for staff now rather than trying to address later the consequences of staff burnout and high attrition rates. The incentive involves Wobble rooms set up to care for those who care (Rimmer 2020). In essence, these are drop-in rooms stocked with drinks, food and treats. Staff can leave messages of support for each other and there are also guided sessions with psychological input from trained facilitators. Assistance is also available virtually if staff are off site. The project has been positively evaluated with many areas considering holding on to these spaces permanently.

Schwartz Rounds

Another well-being initiative also seeks to create a supportive space for staff to come together (Maben et al. 2021). Established first in America and introduced into the UK in 2009, Schwartz Rounds were originally inspired by healthcare lawyer, Kenneth

Schwartz. Whilst undergoing end-of-life care he recognised that small acts of kindness make the unbearable bearable: 'It was the being cared about rather than cared for that made the difference' (Schwartz 1995). He also realised that stress often has a negative impact on staff triggering psychological distress which in turn can lead to burnout.

Schwartz Rounds were established through the Schwartz Centre for Compassionate Care (SCCC), a non-profit organisation set up to develop and implement the approach across the healthcare sector. The Rounds were licenced and introduced into the UK and Ireland by the Point of Care Foundation attracting over two hundred subscriptions from organisations by 2017 (Point of Care Foundation 2017). Their purpose is to help staff to reconnect with the initial motivation and core values which first drew them to a career in healthcare. A structured time and place provide an opportunity to reflect on the emotional impacts of their working day. No clinical solutions or suggestions are offered. The aim is simply for a safe place so that staff feel able to communicate and seek support, thereby enhancing well-being and enabling them to better care for their patients. One of our recent community-based students recognised that personal resilience interlinks crucially with the health of the whole team.

Reflective Extract

Stress and anxiety are a widespread issue within the NHS, so it is important to look at supporting and caring for all my colleagues whatever their roles are within the surgery. At present there does not appear to be any formal way of discussing people's thoughts, feelings and concerns apart from annual appraisals and an individual seeking support for themselves. During my research I have come across the RCN's 'Healthy workplace, Healthy you' tool kit and guidelines and feel that this may be something I could discuss at my place of work in the hope it may be adopted. I plan to discuss this at our next staff meeting as this could be an ideal way of starting to build awareness and giving support to each other.

Talking things through with a colleague or supervisor can be very helpful in coming to terms with difficult events. Another returner reflected on how vulnerable she felt when confronted by relatives angry to find their father (a patient suffering with dementia) distressed and uncomfortable having just evacuated his bowels incontinently. She was able to calm the situation and demonstrate to the family that the care was not sub-standard. What helped her most, however, was the emotional support that came quickly from the sister in charge and the wider team whose shared experiences helped her recover self-esteem.

Talking things through with a colleague or supervisor can be very helpful in coming to terms with difficult events. Occasionally situations are so emotionally draining that some quiet reflective time is needed to validate and process feelings. This is when a journal can be therapeutic. Once emotions are expressed in writing they often feel more manageable, bringing reassurance and enabling insight. As you move on through your first few weeks back in practice and start to feel more confident, it is good to mark your progress by looking back on those early, perhaps more apprehensive journal entries (Tate 2013). During practice brief notes or key phrases are all that is needed, and all that time is likely to allow. Too much introspection can be counterproductive, especially in the early days when self-doubt may surface. It is important to find a balance. Whilst writing things down can help us to de-stress and off-load, some may prefer phone audio notes or even pictures or doodles which help to make sense of challenging experiences. Revisiting these records when we are less emotionally involved can be enlightening.

Extract from a Reflective Account

I feel that awareness of what triggers my stress is key to managing it in the future so keeping a reflective journal will enable me to identify common themes. Scammell (2017) and Hart et al. (2017) both conclude that critical reflection is the essence of building resilience in nurses. By using a reflective journal, I also hope that this will encourage me to look at self-care and being kind to myself.

Scammell J (2017) Resilience in the Workplace: Personal and Organisational Factors. *British Journal of Nursing.* 26(16): 939

Hart P, Brannan J, De Chesnay (2012) Resilience in Nurses: An Integrative Review. *Journal of Nursing Management.* 22(6): 720–734

COMPASSION

A dear nursing friend once took time to explain the roots of the meaning of the word 'compassion'. She said that it comes from the Latin *'pati'* which means 'to suffer'; and the prefix 'com' means 'with'. When we feel compassion for another, we are suffering with them. For a person's job to involve willingly suffering with others is therefore a huge undertaking, a great privilege, but also a weighty burden. Yet this is exactly what nurses do day after day. Not only is it written into our professional standards of practice and behaviour (NMC 2018a) but, arguably, it is given the most prominence, coming as it does within the first line of the NMC Code. We must:

> '1 Treat people as individuals and uphold their dignity.
> To achieve this, you must:
> 1.1 treat people with kindness, respect and compassion.'
>
> (NMC 2018a)

This first section of the Code centres on the need to prioritise people, putting the needs and interests of others before ourselves. When we see what happens in its absence, we are reminded of the absolute necessity of this intrinsic human quality in our work. Yet, compassion is complicated. Clarifying and promoting this concept within healthcare practice and educational contexts is challenging (Schantz 2007; Bramley and Milika 2014; Curtis 2014). For Dewar and Christley (2013) compassion is about recognising and responding to vulnerability as well as suffering.

Halifax (2014) developed a process to support nurses in not just 'caring for' but 'caring about' patients, echoing the earlier words of Kenneth Schwartz. This is compassionate care, defined by the almost invisible small touches of thoughtfulness which matter profoundly to patients and families and may leave the giver with a warm glow (Pearson 2006). These kind and gentle acts are perhaps what motivated us to follow a career in nursing, yet only when they become absent from care do they seem to carry weight at management level. Halifax (2014) acknowledges that nursing's best asset is at risk of being lost in the stressful environment in which we work. She suggests the use of the mnemonic, GRACE, to help bring focus and clarity to our interactions with patients, thus developing the therapeutic compassionate relationship. GRACE acts as a reminder to pause and attend. Not only do these simple steps relate to compassion, but they also promote mindfulness, encouraging us to ground ourselves before we engage.

G *ground yourself – pause, think, feel your feet on the ground, take a few seconds to gather yourself.*

R *recall intention .... purpose.*

A *attune first to yourself; acknowledging how we feel can help us to refocus and give unbiased attention.*

C *consider what will serve. What is needed here?*

E *engage and mark the end, so you can move forward without ruminating: this can inhibit the next encounter.*

(Halifax 2014)

Again, though compassion must start with the self. It is suggested that self-compassion can help us to strengthen our emotional resilience (Durkin et al. 2016; Kotera et al. 2020). Being kind and gentle to ourselves helps to stop the onslaught of undue self-criticism when things fall short of expectations. The concept of self-compassion is found in Buddhist thinking and embraces mindfulness, a sense of shared humanity and self-understanding (Neff 2009). It may feel like another buzzword, but self-compassion conveys urgent truths to those who care for others. When juggling many demands, we must be realistic about what is doable and not judge ourselves harshly when things go wrong. Imperfection is a quality shared by us all – a compassionate outlook brings us all together. In the following account one of our returning students shares an experience from her practice placement. Her reflections lead her to conclude that caring for self and others are intertwined.

Returner's Account

The practice nurses in the surgery see patients in two sessions each day. As part of my practice placement, it was decided that I would conduct my own small session under the supervision of my Practice Assessor. Four patients were due to attend for leg ulcer dressings, with each patient allocated a time suitable for their dressing needs. Nurse sessions at the surgery are in 15-minute sections and can be adjusted depending on the needs of the patient. The first session went as planned but then the subsequent session overran because the dressings were new to me and took longer than I expected. This then led to the last two appointments running late and the patients having to wait and potentially being inconvenienced. My role was to provide quality nursing care in a timely manner. I felt that I did not achieve this and consequently this made me feel inadequate and have negative thoughts about myself. This internal dialogue included feelings such as not being good enough, worrying what colleagues/patients were thinking about me and whether I would ever manage to run a clinic independently on time.

It is vitally important that staff, including myself, are aware of how our own health affects patient care. Stress and anxiety in my previous nursing post was one of the main reasons that I took a career break. Stress was a daily occurrence and I remember having similar thoughts and feelings then; to prevent experiencing burnout again I really want to be able to deal with these feelings in a more positive manner. Schwabe and Wolf (2009) suggest that the reaction to stress is more likely to be habit-based rather than a cognitive behaviour and this may suggest why I reacted the way I did to this situation – it was a learnt response from my previous experiences. During my career break I undertook personal counselling and mindfulness training to help me to identify issues that have perhaps influenced me and the way I approach life. Mindfulness is the practice of being present in the moment, developing skills in acceptance, attention and awareness (White 2014). White believes that being mindful can enable care to become more holistic in nature which can only be of benefit to patients and practitioners alike. Van der Riet et al. (2014) showed in their research that this approach not only helped to improve self-awareness in a group of student nurses but it also reduced negative internal dialogue and feelings. In this instance, however, I think my old learnt habits just came straight to the fore – they just took over, perhaps because I was not expecting to have this reaction to the events. In retrospect I think I should have given more thought to the possibility that I would return to feeling negative in stressful situations. If I had done this, I may have been able to identify what was happening quicker, take a step back and reflect on how to best manage the situation. I sometimes feel that I set myself very high standards and if I do not achieve these, I am letting myself down and other people – patients and colleagues. In this situation I felt I was letting down the patients who were having to wait and my colleagues because I had to ask for help. I think that this shows that I can have unrealistic expectations of what I can achieve as in this situation and on reflection, I do not think that it could have turned out any differently unless the caseload had been undertaken by a more experienced team member.

There are high levels of stress in all sectors of the NHS (NHS Employers 2019). It can often seem that everyone else is managing and it's just yourself floundering, so I think that it is important to check how colleagues are feeling and acknowledge to them how you are feeling. Nurses know the importance of the 6Cs (Care, Compassion, Competence, Communication, Courage, Commitment) (NHS England 2015) necessary to give compassionate care to patients, but I feel that this should be applied not only to patients but also to ourselves as nurses. If we cannot care for ourselves, we could potentially struggle to deliver high-quality care to our patients.

On a practical level, I feel that initially I may need slightly longer appointment times with patients until I have gained more experience. This will allow time for reflection immediately after the episode of care and time to catch up if I'm running behind. I could also ask for patients in the waiting room to be informed by the reception team of any delays so that they are fully informed that an issue has arisen, and they may be seen late.

In conclusion, I have gained insight into how a clinic runs and understand that clinics can easily be thrown off course by unexpected events. I feel that as my practice develops, I will become more proficient at managing my time. This reflection has enabled me to realise that I am still relatively new to practice nursing and that I need to be kinder to myself and ask for assistance and offer support to others.

COMPASSION FATIGUE

You may identify with this returner's concerns, perhaps also having experienced high levels of workplace stress which eventually led you to leave the profession. The flip side of compassionate care is compassion fatigue which has been likened to post-traumatic stress disorder (Figley 2002). The term has no standard universal definition but is often used when referring to the experiences of healthcare staff. Put simply, it is viewed as the cost of caring, and in looser terms refers to the inability to respond to a request for help because physical and emotional exhaustion means there is no more to give (Moore et al. 2021).

Compassion fatigue can undermine our well-being leading to symptoms such as insomnia, anxiety, fatigue, irritation, loss of interest, boredom and, unsurprisingly, a loss of compassion (Quinal et al. 2009; Boyle 2011). As a form of self-preservation, healthcare workers become detached and remote from the caring aspect of nursing, delivering task-orientated care without emotional involvement. Sadly, compassion fatigue is a reality that is associated with repeated stresses within the work environment. Nurses are expected to manage their feelings and behave in a professional manner whatever challenges they face. This can be very difficult when trying to provide care that is empathetic and compassionate.

You may have witnessed or encountered experiences of compassion fatigue in your own practice. If this was one of the reasons prompting you to step back from the nursing profession, you will not be alone. It is important to take stock of this on your return journey.

BURNOUT

Sometimes viewed as the ultimate consequence of compassion fatigue, the term 'burnout' was first coined in the 1970s (Freudenberger 1974) and then explored further by Maslach (2003) who identified it as a state of emotional exhaustion predominantly resulting from excessive work stress. Maslach devised a measurement scale called the Maslach Burnout Inventory (MBI) which is still widely in use today and continues to endorse the fact that the three key indicators for burnout are emotional exhaustion, depersonalisation, and reduced personal accomplishment. In their comprehensive review of the literature, Dall'Ora et al. (2020) find accord with Maslach, agreeing that the strongest factors linked to burnout in nursing are heavy workloads, long shifts with little flexibility, time pressures, low staffing levels and high psychological demands, poor leadership and a sense of low control.

In an interesting report by Health Education England (HEE) the suggestion is made that the very personality traits often attributed to, and indeed deemed as estimable, in healthcare professionals are the same that make them especially vulnerable to burnout (HEE 2014a). These include altruistic qualities such as self-giving, empathy, not recognising personal limits and extreme conscientiousness. Again, this is echoed in The People Plan, which confirms that 'those in caring roles often wait until they are very unwell before raising their hand' (NHS England 2020). Some authors of the subject view a decline into burnout more as a process which charts a descent over time. If we imagine a downward line of travel from compassionate caring commitment to something much more negative, we can see how some of the signs of burnout – indifference, cynicism, feelings of helplessness and absenteeism – would appear at the other end of such a continuum.

Delgado et al. (2017) suggest that a dissonance arises within nurses when they must repeatedly suppress their own feelings of distress or anxiety whilst outwardly behaving calm and professional. This conflict can lead to nursing burnout, made clear in the Francis inquiry which also identified institutional, political and social elements as major contributory factors (House of Commons Select Committee 2018). However, Labrague et al. (2017) point out that organisations can also guard against burnout.

This is a reminder again to check the ethos of your future employer as well as just the local working conditions.

It is crucial for healthcare workers to acknowledge that their emotional health is a factor in providing good quality care. Opportunities to debrief have long been recognised as strategies beneficial in providing emotional first aid (Neil et al. 1974). Support from empathetic peers and colleagues may be mutually beneficial and can provide effective protection against the hazards of a stressful work environment. In addition, strong friendships and family relationships may help to boost self-esteem and emotional security (McDonald et al. 2016).

BALANCE

In the context of well-being, balance is explained as the flow of energy that sustains giving and receiving (RCN 2021a). It will be determined by the choices you make throughout your return journey. Notwithstanding the inevitable stresses and pinch points that come with most focused endeavours, try to work out from the start what feels balanced for you. What are your weekly commitments? Where are your priorities – both personal and general – and what could be reviewed, postponed or delegated to others? You will need to keep at least two days per week free for your practice hours (some courses will require more), and you will also need to set time aside for study. Good planning and support structures will provide some ballast and alleviate stress and anxiety. Being familiar with what is expected of you also helps, although this may be difficult prior to starting the programme. However, course dates are usually identified from an early stage which can help with managing other responsibilities such as part-time work and childcare.

Towards the end of the course, you may feel the weight of impending academic assessments, and there may still be some proficiencies to achieve in your practice placement. Balance is also about pacing so try to plan these last few weeks. Extensions to assignment deadlines are usually granted in the face of specific difficulties, and placement lengths can often be adjusted slightly to enable successful completion. You may have young children, teenagers or partners who are not all together happy with your current new routines. Although it may feel easier just to get things done, it is important to share responsibilities. You will need time and energy to achieve your goal, and this may involve compromises. There may be areas in your life that you may have to relinquish for someone else to take on. Receiving as well as giving may require you to accept things done differently. This is not always easy, but it can activate others and it will save you precious time.

Balance can come in the shape of exchanging thoughts and ideas, using social support networks as sounding boards and to maintain perspective. Post COVID-19 pandemic, COPE Scotland have developed a resource booklet 'You matter too' in support of the well-being of healthcare professionals (COPE Scotland 2021). It provides insight into the art and therapeutic value of communication. One simple chat with another person can have a huge impact. Often, we can fix our own problems, but just need another person to validate our feelings first. COPE Scotland (2021) suggests that 'kinder conversations build a kinder world'. Although this may sound simplistic, it has a powerful resonance.

In Chapter 4 we introduced the notion of three buckets (Reason 2004) to help assess our vulnerability to risky situations in practice. Here comes another bucket shown in Figure 6.1 which has a similar application. It was originally conceived by Brabban and Turkinton (2002) and has since been reproduced by many (including Mental Health UK) to show personal stress levels and how we manage them. The first thing to note about your bucket is its size. Those with a sensitivity to stress may have a larger bucket than those whose temperament or strategies enable them to cope reasonably well. You will notice that low down on the side of the bucket there is a tap. Stress flows into the bucket and the tap is positioned to open and let it out to maintain good coping levels. If the tap is not working well, however, the stress levels in the bucket will rise and may threaten to overflow.

Stress hormones such as cortisol and adrenaline are constantly with us, not just helping us to fight, flight or freeze in an emergency, but also (in smaller measures) spurring us through our daily tasks. However, when life becomes busier with the added pressures of working to an assignment deadline or feeling scrutinised in practice, these natural chemicals may stay uncomfortably raised for protracted periods of time, and then we can start to feel overwhelmed.

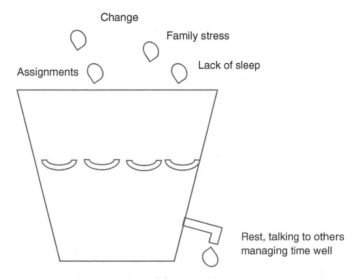

FIGURE 6.1 Stress bucket. *Source:* Adapted from Brabban and Turkinton 2002.

Common signs of stress include fatigue, irritability, not feeling quite yourself, anxiety and feeling isolated, insomnia, lack of appetite and a sense of your heart pounding or racing. Self-awareness helps us to perceive and understand our individual responses to stress so that we can recognise difficult days and re-balance accordingly. Stress hormones can be calmed and regulated through healthy diet, good hydration and exercise. Try to develop positive activities that will mitigate the effects of stress: hobbies, social events and just being outside can all be beneficial. Taking time to regroup, rest and relax will help maintain motivation, perspective and a refocusing of goals and objectives. For some, a structured and proactive approach can be useful; this might involve listing identified stressors such as a limited support network or episodes of poor health alongside helpful actions such as talking to others or requesting an extension for an academic assignment. In summary, the aim is to manage our stress buckets so that times of challenge are balanced and levelled by good coping strategies.

When asked about what keeps them well, one of our recent Return to Practice cohorts had some simple and straightforward answers which we have captured in the mind map shown in Figure 6.2. Their message supports the view that well-being is sustained in a variety of ways. Maintaining connections and relaxing with others is crucial, coupled with care of the physical self. As we have seen from the literature, positive working environments matter, and of course this points to an area about which we have less control. However, we can conclude that actively balancing a range of activities and strategies is the best way to keep ourselves well and happy.

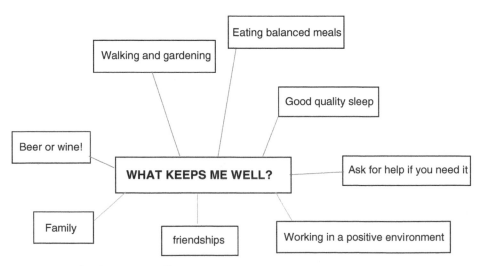

FIGURE 6.2   What keeps me well.

REFERENCES

Aburn, G., Gott, M., and Hoare, K. (2016). What is resilience? An integrative review of the empirical literature. *Journal of Advanced Nursing* 72 (5): 980–1000.

Adan, A. (2012). Cognitive performance and dehydration. *Journal of the American College of Nutrition* 31 (2): 71–78.

Barratt, C. and Wagstaffe, T. (2018). Nursing and mindfulness. In: *Coping and Thriving in Nursing: An Essential Guide for Practice* (ed. P.J. Martin), 62–80. London: SAGE Publications.

Beddoe, L., Davys, A., and Adamson, C. (2013). Educating resilient practitioners. *Social Work Education* 32 (1): 100–117.

Bolton, G. (2010). *Reflective Practice Writing and Professional Development*. London: Sage.

Bolton, G. and Delderfield, R. (2018). *Reflective Practice: Writing and Professional Development*, 5e.

Boyle, D.A. (2011). Countering compassion fatigue: a requisite nursing agenda. *The Online Journal of Issues in Nursing* 16 (1).

Brabban, A. and Turkinton, D. (2002). The search for meaning: detecting congruence between life events, underlying schema and psychotic symptoms. In: *A Casebook of Cognitive Therapy for Psychosis* (ed. A.P. Morrison). Brunner-Routledge.

Bramley, L. and Milika, M. (2014). How does it really feel to be in my shoes? Patients' experiences of compassion within nursing care and their perceptions of developing compassionate nurses. *Journal of Clinical Nursing* 23: 2790–2799. John Wiley & Sons Ltd.

Burton, A., Burgess, C., Dean, S. et al. (2016). How effective are mindfulness-based interventions for reducing stress among healthcare professionals? A systematic review and meta-analysis. *Stress and Health* 33 (1): 3–13. ISSN 1532-3005.

Burton, K., Golding, M., and Griffiths, C. (2011). Barriers to learning for mature students studying HE in an FE college. *Journal of Further and Higher Education* 35 (1): 25–36.

Caruso, D., Masci, I., Cipollone, G., and Palagini, L. (2019). Insomnia and depressive symptoms during the menopausal transition: theoretical and therapeutic implications of a self-reinforcing feedback loop. *Maturitas* 123: 78–81.

Cheng, S.T., Tsui, P.K., and Lam, J.H. (2015). Improving mental health in health care practitioners: randomized controlled trial of a gratitude intervention. *Journal of Consulting and Clinical Psychology* 83 (1): 177–186.

Coates, M. and MacFayden, A. (2021). Student experiences of a return to practice programme: a qualitative study. *British Journal of Nursing* 30 (15): 900–908.

Cope, A. (2017). *Art of Being Brilliant*. Capstone publishers.

COPE Scotland (2021). https://www.cope-scotland.org.

Cope, V., Jones, B., and Hendricks, J. (2016). Why nurses chose to remain in the workforce: portraits of resilience. *Collegian* 23 (1): 87–95.

Csikszentmihalyi, M. (2002). *Flow. The Classic Work on How to Achieve Happiness*. Rider. The Random House Group Limited.

Curtis, K. (2014). Learning the requirements for compassionate practice: student vulnerability and courage. *Nursing Ethics* 21 (2): 210–223.

Dall'Ora, C., Ball, J., Reinius, M., and Griffiths, P. (2020). Burnout in nursing: a theoretical review. *Human Resources for Health* 5; 18 (1): 41.

Davies, N. (2020). Cultivating resilience as a nurse. https://www.independentnurse.co.uk/professional-article/cultivating-resilience-as-a-nurse/215034.

Delgado, C., Upton, D., Ranse, K. et al. (2017). Nurses' resilience and the emotional labour of nursing work: an integrative review of empirical literature. *International Journal of Nursing Studies* 70: 71–88.

Dewar, B. and Christley, Y. (2013). A critical analysis of compassion in practice. *Nursing Standard* 28 (10).

Durkin, M., Beaumont, E., Hollins Martin, C.J., and Carson, J. (2016). A pilot study exploring the relationship between self-compassion, self-judgement, self-kindness, compassion, professional quality of life and wellbeing among UK community nurses. *Nurse Education Today* 46: 109–114.

Eanes, L. (2015). The potential effects of sleep loss on a nurse's health. *American Journal of Nursing* 115 (4): 34–40.

Figley, C. (ed.) (2002). *Treating Compassion Fatigue*. New York: Brunner Routledge.

Foureur, M., Besley, K., Burton, G. et al. (2013). Enhancing the resilience of nurses and midwives: pilot of a mindfulness-based program for increased health, sense of coherence and decreased depression, anxiety, and stress. *Contemporary Nurse* 45 (1): 114–125.

Fox, B.H., Perez, N., Cass, E. et al. (2015). Trauma changes everything: examining the relationship between adverse childhood experiences and serious, violent and chronic juvenile offenders. *Child Abuse & Neglect* 46: 163–173.

Francis, R. (2015). *Freedom to Speak Up: An Independent Review into Creating an Open and Honest Reporting Culture in the NHS*. London: The Stationary Office.

Free Dictionary. (n.d.) https://www.thefreedictionary.com.

Freudenberger, H.J. (1974). Staff burn-out. *Journal of Social Issues* 30 (1): 159–165.

Funning (2010 May). *Spirituality: RCN Bulletin*.

Galderisi, S., Heinz, A., Kastrup, M. et al. (2015). Toward a new definition of mental health. *World Psychiatry* 14 (2): 231–233.

Gandy, J. (2012). First findings of the United Kingdom fluid intake study. *Nutrition Today* 47: S14–S16.

Grant, C., Wallace, L., and Spurgeon, P. (2013). An exploration of the psychological factors affecting remote e-workers job effectiveness, well-being and work-life balance. *Employee Relations* 35 (5): 527–546.

Halifax, J. (2014). G.R.A.C.E. for nurses: cultivating compassion in nurse/patient interactions. *Journal of Nursing Education and Practice* 4 (1): 121–128.

Hart, P.L., Brannan, J.D., and De Chesnay, M. (2014). Resilience in nurses: an integrative review. *Journal of Nursing Management* 22 (6): 720–734.

Health Education England (2014). *Growing Nursing Numbers: Literature Review on Nurses Leaving the NHS*. London: HEE.

Henning, S.M., Yang, J., Shao, P. et al. (2017). Health benefit of vegetable/fruit juice-based diet: role of microbiome. *Scientific Reports* 7: 2167.

Henshall, C., Davey, Z., and Jackson, D. (2020). Nursing resilience interventions-A way forward in challenging healthcare territories. *Journal of Clinical Nursing* 29 (19–20): 3597–3599.

Hochschild, A.R. (1983). *The Managed Heart: Commercialization of Human Feeling.* Berkeley, CA: University of California Press.

House of Commons Select Committee (2018). https://publications.parliament.uk/pa/cm201719/cmselect/cmhealth/353/35302.htm.

Hulatt, I. (2019). The toll emotional labour is taking on nurses' mental health. *Nursing Standard* 34 (11): 41.

Kinnair, D. (2020). *No medals, badges or claps this time – just pay nursing staff fairly.* Cited in Manthorpe J, Iliffe S, Gillen P, et al. (2022) Clapping for carers in the Covid-19 crisis: Carers' reflections in a UK survey. *Health Soc Care Community* 30:1442–1449. https://doi.org/10.1111/hsc.13474.

Kitchener, B.A. and Jorm, A.F. (2008). Mental health first aid: an international programme for early intervention. *Early Intervention in Psychiatry* 2: 55–61.

Kotera, Y., Green, P., and Sheffield, D. (2020). Work-life balance of UK construction workers: relationship with mental health. *Construction Management and Economics* 38 (3): 291–303.

Labrague, L.J., McEnroe-Petitte, D.M., Gloe, D. et al. (2017). Organizational politics, nurses' stress, burnout levels, turnover intention, and job satisfaction. *International Nursing Review* 64 (1): 109–116.

Ma, X., Yue, Z.Q., Gong, Z.Q. et al. (2017). The effect of diaphragmatic breathing on attention, negative affect, and stress in healthy adults. *Frontiers in Psychology* 8: 874.

Maben, J., Taylor, C., Reynolds, E. et al. (2021). Realist evaluation of Schwartz rounds® for enhancing the delivery of compassionate healthcare: understanding how they work, for whom, and in what contexts. *BMC Health Services Research* 18; 21 (1): 709.

Martin, C.M. (2018). Resilience and health(care): a dynamic adaptive perspective. *Journal of Evaluation in Clinical Practice* 24: 1319–1322.

Masento, N.A., Golightly, M., Field, D.T. et al. (2014). Effects of hydration status on cognitive performance and mood. *British Journal of Nutrition* 111 (10): 1841–1852.

Maslach, C. (2003). *Burnout: The Cost of Caring.* Cambridge, MA: Malor Books.

McCraty, R. and Childre, D. (2004). The grateful heart: the psychophysiology of appreciation. In: *Series in Affective Science. The Psychology of Gratitude* (ed. R.A. Emmons and M.E. McCullough), 230–255. New York: Oxford University press.

McDonald, G., Jackson, D., Vickers, M.H., and Wilkes, L. (2016). Surviving workplace adversity: a qualitative study of nurses and midwives and their strategies to increase personal resilience. *Journal of Nursing Management* 24 (1): 123–131.

Mental Health First Aid England (MHFA) (2019). Impact report 2018-2019. https://mhfaengland.org/mhfa-centre/impact-report-2019.pdf.

Menzies, I.E.P. (1960). A case-study in the functioning of social systems as a defence against anxiety: a report on a study of the nursing service of a general hospital. *Human*

Relations 13: 95–121. In: Smith, P. (2012). *The Emotional Labour of Nursing Revisited: Can Nurses Still Care?* 2e. Palgrave Macmillan.

Moore, M.F., Montgomery, L., and Cobbs, T. (2021). Increasing student success through in-class resilience education. *Nurse Education in Practice* 50: 102948.

Neff, K.D. (2009). The role of self-compassion in development: a healthier way to relate to oneself. *Human Development* 52 (4): 211–214.

Neil, T., Oney, J., Difonso, L. et al. (1974). *Emotional First Aid.* Louisville, KY: Kemper-Behavioural Sciences Associates.

NHS England (2015). Introducing the 6C's. *NHS England.* [online]. Available from: https://www.england.nhs.uk/6cs/wp-content/uploads/sites/25/2015/03/introducing-the-6cs.pdf.

NHS Employers (2019) Stress and its Impact on the work place. *NHS Employers* [online]. Available from: https://www.nhsemployers.org/retention-and-staff-experience/health-and-wellbeing/taking-a-targeted-approach/taking-a-targeted-approach/stress-and-its-impact-on-the-workplace.

The NHS Constitution NHS England (2021). London. DH. https://www.gov.uk/government/publications/the-nhs-constitution-for-england.

NHS Digital (2022). *NHS vacancy statistics England april 2015 – june 2021 experimental statistics.* https://digital.nhs.uk/data-and-information/publications/statistical/nhs-vacancies-survey/april-2015---march-2021.

NHS England (2020). We are the NHS: people plan 2020/21. https://www.england.nhs.uk/ournhspeople/online-version.

NMC (2018a). *The Code. Professional Standards of Practice and Behaviour for Nurses, Midwives, and Nursing Associates.* London: NMC.

NMC (2018b). *Future Nurse: Standards of Proficiency for Registered Nurses.* London: NMC.

NMC (2020). The NMC register 1 April 2019 – 31 March 2020. https://www.nmc.org.uk/globalassets/sitedocuments/nmcregister/march-2020/nmc-register-march-2020.pdf.

NMC (2022). *The Professional Duty of Candour.* London: NMC.

Pearson, A. (2006). Powerful caring. *Nursing Standard* 20 (948): 20–22.

Pietroni, P. (1986). *Holistic Living.* J M Dent & Sons Ltd.

Point of Care Foundation (2017). Schwartz rounds. Available at: www.pointofcarefoundation.org.uk/our-work/schwartz-rounds.

Quinal, L., Harford, S., and Rutledge, D.N. (2009). Secondary traumatization in oncology staff. *Cancer Nursing* 32 (4): E1E7.

RCN (2010). *Guidance on Safe Nurse Staffing Levels in UK.* London: Royal College of Nursing.

RCN (2015) Healthy Workplace, Healthy You. *RCN* [online]. Available from: https://www.rcn.org.uk/healthy-workplace/get-started

RCN (2020). *Building a better future*. https://www.rcn.org.uk/professional-development/publications/rcn-builiding-a-better-future-covid-pub-009366#detailTab.

RCN (2021a). Healthy workplace toolkit. https://www.rcn.org.uk/healthy-workplace/healthy-workplaces.

Reason, J. (2004). Beyond the organisational accident: the need for 'error wisdom' on the frontline. *Quality & Safety in Health Care* 13 (Supplement 2): ii28–i33.

Rimmer, A. (2020). Sixty seconds on …wobble rooms. *British Medical Journal* doi: 10.1136/bmj.m4461.

Roper, N., Logan, W., and Tierney, A. (1980). *The Elements of Nursing*. Edinburgh: Churchill Livingstone.

Roy, C. (1980). The Roy Adaptation Model. In: *Conceptual Models for Nursing Practice*, 2e (ed. J.P. Riehl and C. Roy), 179–188. Norwalk, Connecticut: Appleton-Century-Crofts.

Schantz, M. (2007). Compassion a concept analysis. *Nursing Forum* 42: 48–55.

Schwabe, L. and Wolf, O. (2009) Stress Prompts Habit behaviour in Humans. *The Journal of Neuroscience*. 29 (22): 7191–7198

Schwartz, K. (1995). A patient's story. Boston Globe Magazine. https://www.theschwartzcenter.org/members/media/patients_story.pdf.

Smith, P. (1992). *The Emotional Labour of Nursing: Its Impact on Interpersonal Relations, Management and Educational Environment*. Bloomsbury Publishing.

Smith, P. and Gray, B. (2001). Emotional labour of nursing revisited: caring and Learning 2000. *Nurse Education in Practice* 1 (1): 42–49.

Sun, N., Wei, L., Shi, S. et al. (2020). A qualitative study on the psychological experience of caregivers of COVID-19 patients. *American Journal of Infection Control* 48 (6): 592–598.

Tate, S. (2013). Writing to learn, writing reflectively. In: *Reflective Practice in Nursing*, 5e (ed. C. Bulman and S. Schutz). Wiley-Blackwell.

Tennant, R., Hiller, L., Fishwick, R. et al. (2007). The Warwick-Edinburgh Mental Well-being Scale (WEMWBS): development and UK validation. *Health and Quality of Life Outcomes* 5: 63.

Trueland, J. (2017). Resilience is not about trying harder. *Nursing Standard* 32 (24): 18–20.

Trueland, J. (2022). Weight loss support for nurses: apps and healthy food options. *Nursing Standard* 37 (8): 70–73.

Turner, K. (2009). Mindfulness: the present moment in clinical social work. *Clinical Social Work Journal* 37 (2): 95–103.

Van der Reit, P., Rossiter, R., Kirby, D., Dluzewka, T., and Hartman, C. (2014). Piloting a stress management program for undergraduate nursing students: student feedback and lesson learned. *Nurse Education Today* 35 (1): 44–49.

White, L. (2014). Mindfulness in nursing: an evolutionary concept analysis. *Journal of Advanced Nursing* 70 (2): 282–294.

Witkoski, A. and Dickson, V. (2010). Hospital staff nurses' work hours, meal periods, and rest breaks. A review from an occupational health nurse perspective. *AAOHN Journal* 58 (11): 489–497.

World Health Organisation (2022). Mental health: strengthening our response. https://www.who.int/news-room/fact-sheets/detail/mental-health-strengthening-our-response#:~:text=Mental%20health%20is%20a%20state,and%20contribute%20to%20their%20community.

Wysong, P.R. and Driver, E. (2009). Patients' perceptions of nurses' skill. *Critical Care Nurse* 29: 24–37.

Xie, Z., Wang, A., and Chen, B. (2011). Nurse burnout and its association with occupational stress in a cross-sectional study in Shanghai. *Journal of Advanced Nursing* 67: 1537–1546.

CHAPTER 7

Returning to Study

Returning to nursing practice also involves a return to study. This may be a daunting prospect. Indeed, many returners express as much anxiety at the thought of writing assignments as they do about stepping back into clinical settings. Courses tutors understand these concerns and are experienced at offering reassurance and support.

Before commencing a Return to Practice course, it is a good idea to think through how you feel about studying again. It may be that your last experience of academic work was recent and positive and therefore you are comfortable about your skills in this area, or you may have more negative associations due perhaps to not receiving sufficient support in the past or recalling difficulties with certain types of assessment. For example, a common worry for many returners is being tested on their numeracy. Maths anxiety is felt by many in the general population (Chinn 2012). Chinn's research shows that fear of maths can start at school where individuals learn to avoid sums rather than face the sense of failure and low self-esteem triggered by not finding the right answer. Obstacles such as these can persist, undermining our confidence as adult learners (Canning 2010). Becoming a student again is likely to invoke a range of emotions. It is important to acknowledge these as they will help signal areas of strength and limitation, providing good indicators of where best to focus your attention.

Returning to Nursing Practice: Confidence and Competence, First Edition. Ros Wray and Mary Kitson.
© 2023 John Wiley & Sons Ltd. Published 2023 by John Wiley & Sons Ltd.

Here are some comments from recent Return to Practice students about their experiences of studying again:

Words of Wisdom

It's hard to blow out the academic cobwebs – do your first written account early so you can use the rest of your time at full function!

It takes time to feel confident about studying again, but as you refresh your knowledge your confidence increases.

It is surprising how much you are capable of.

I had not forgotten everything! Old skills do resurface!

I enjoyed the academic side of the course, and I felt a sense of achievement on completing the assignments.

I need to have more confidence in my own abilities.

The life skills I have learnt during my career break have been very valuable.

The final two comments are especially significant. Returning nurses are nearly always mature adult learners and some, as already noted, may be entering university education for the first time. They can possess what Race (2001) calls 'unconscious competence', meaning that they may be unaware of the educational worth of their existing skills and life experience. Navarre Cleary (2012) has also written about this subject, pointing out that adult learners often feel more anxious about completing assignments than students who have entered higher education straight from school or college. Once this lack of confidence is turned around, there often blossoms in its place an excitement and appetite for future study.

PREPARATION

In Chapter 3 we stressed the importance of self-assessment as part of the preparation for a return to nursing practice. For study too, it is vital to weigh up your current position and the way ahead. Perhaps the first two questions to ask yourself is what can I do well, and what will I need help with. The answers will provide counterpoints from which you can explore other areas. For example, a positive aspect may be that you have good childcare arrangements ensuring quiet evenings and some weekends in which to study. On the more negative side, however, you may be worried about writing assignments because it is fifteen years since you were last in education. Having identified a point of concern the next step is to investigate further. Is this a generalised sense of feeling rusty and out-of-date, or is it related specifically to past difficulties with essay writing or referencing? Do you see yourself as a nurse whose strength is practice rather than academic study? As we have discussed in earlier chapters, self-assessment is about recognising your strengths and acknowledging areas for future development. Understandably, you may feel disinclined to commence this activity because it feels hard to pinpoint and may provoke some anxieties. However, although the activity can be arduous, once completed it can be very helpful, enabling a student to see the full picture with specific goals clearly set out and existing skills and abilities affirmed.

Aside from course documentation, one useful preparatory tool to have in your armoury is mind mapping, and we would recommend this approach when you need to know quickly the breadth and scale of a project, be it an academic assignment or a personal plan of action. Mind mapping promotes creative free thinking and a structure to illuminate patterns and connections (Buzan 2018). We hope that the mind map in Figure 7.1 will provide a good introduction to study skills. Some of the key elements identified will be explored further in this chapter.

TIME

Prospective nurse returners are usually very busy people. They are already likely to be balancing a range of other commitments; add in a Return to Practice course and the need for good time management becomes critical to success. Courses tend to be no more than six months in duration, and necessarily pack theory and practice together. This means that you will find yourself completing placement hours, proficiencies and writing about practice experiences all at the same time.

The issue of time is a recurrent and important theme in studying. For nurse returners, it is especially so as the comments below attest. We have therefore devoted a considerable section of this chapter to the topic, and hope that you find these discussions helpful.

Words of Wisdom

It is tricky juggling children, house, work and study, but ultimately satisfying when it is all done!
It is harder this time around because I have a family.
Be organised and prepared! It is not as scary as you think.

Your Body Clock

A person's sense of time starts internally. Our twenty-four-hour cycle of night and day embraces sleep and activity, but the timeframe for these states can vary greatly from one individual to the next. The daily round of work, rest and refreshment are shaped by necessity and routine, but also by our own internal body clock. Where a good breakfast may feel essential for some people, others may prefer not to eat until lunchtime. Sometimes called circadian rhythms, these internal biological patterns are largely inherited and play a part in regulating many of our bodily functions including digestion and hormone levels (Foster and Kreitzman 2017). Disrupting these internal time settings and movements can upset our work–life balance as we all know from

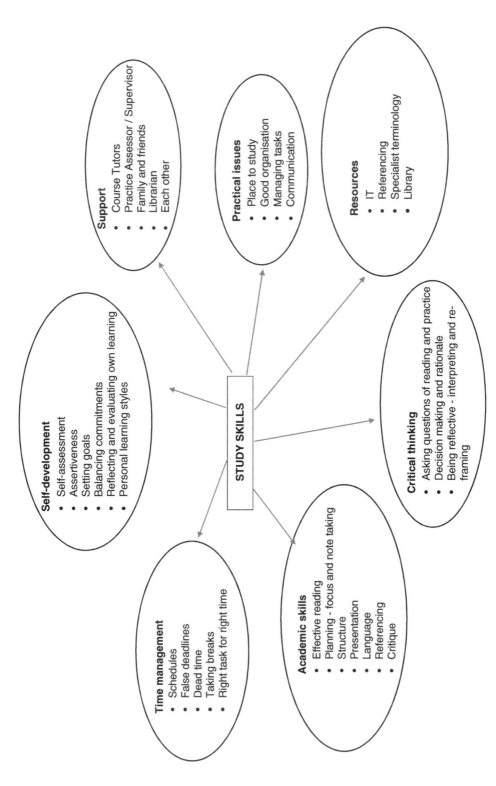

FIGURE 7.1 Mind map of study skills.

experiences of shift work or jet lag. Put simply, we live better if we respect our inner body clock. There is interesting literature on this subject; along with Foster and Kreitzman's (2017) introduction to circadian rhythms, Roenneberg (2012) has also written extensively on internal time and is well worth reading.

When thinking about good times to study, first consider whether you are an early bird or a night owl. You are likely to produce your best academic work when your study time and your internal time are synchronised. Do you naturally feel more alert in the mornings or the evenings? Famous night owls include Charles Darwin and Barack Obama. Famous early birds are Benjamin Franklin and Napoleon.

Of course, it is crucial to factor in your current lifestyle and activities as these may require you to modify your natural timings. If you know that you work best in the mornings but have a young family of early risers, you may find that some study will have to be scheduled for the evenings when your children are in bed. Importantly, save the more demanding study tasks for your preferred time for working. Higher level activities such as academic writing and critiquing research articles will find their best flow when you are in tune with your internal rhythm. Conversely, if you are night owl attempting to start your essay first thing in the morning, you may struggle; far better to use this time for notetaking, or proof-checking draft work.

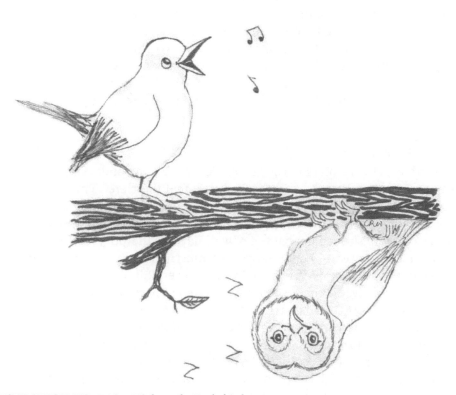

ILLUSTRATION NO. 7.1A Night owl - Early bird.

Schedules and Planners

Once you have identified optimum times for study, you will need to make plans. Mapping out your commitments will enable you to weigh up free periods and pinch points. A schedule that plots each week of the course duration will help you to organise your time. This will come naturally to planners and feel restrictive to those who prefer spontaneity. We would urge you all to use a method of some kind to record your week and study time and communicate this to those in your household. Choose a visible display such as a planner or calendar for others to see – fridges are especially good for this! Being able to balance competing activities and obligations is a challenging task but also one that is fundamental to success. Conspicuous reminders of how busy you are will encourage family and friends to offer timely and thoughtful support, and it will also assist you in maintaining a healthy work–life balance. Factoring in breaks is also essential.

Matching the ups and downs of your typical week to the periods of study time you have scheduled will enable you to decide what you can do when and where. Try to be realistic in your planning. If you care for an elderly relative or have a part-time job or voluntary commitments, you will need to think about how tiredness from one role may impact on your ability to study effectively within the same twenty-four period. It may be better not to study between working days, but instead to count this as much needed rest, aware that you will be fresher for taking some time out. These are all individual decisions that only you can make. The chief thing is to know that whatever your circumstances, you will need to weigh up options and choose what works best for you.

Pacing is crucial. The sheer weight of information delivered in course inductions can trigger a sense of urgency, tipping students into a frenzy of precipitous reading and writing, accompanied by rising nervous energy, and sometimes even catastrophising. To some extent, this 'front-loading' of material is a necessary preparation for practice. However, the reality is that courses are designed to unfold in line with placements; there is no rush, and it can even be counter-productive to try to get ahead before you have had time to settle.

A good tip is to first mark in your schedule any holidays or days off. This does two things: it sends a reassuring signal to loved ones that there are some dates which are sacrosanct; and it will immediately enable you to see the light and shade, the work and play, of the next few months. Next, add in a nominal weekly day off from the course so that you can establish a regular pattern of workdays, be they for practice or study. You will of course also need to honour any remaining non-course activities. Structuring your time in this way can be very beneficial; however, it is also important to preserve some flexibility. As we all know, some days will not go according to plan. More importantly, you will need to be adaptable to accommodate your time to the work patterns of placement supervisors or to possible changes in timetabled course sessions.

When it comes to course submission points, some students find it helpful to work with a false deadline (perhaps a week before the actual date) so that they have contingency for the unexpected. For others, a false deadline ensures that they finish the assignment early, preventing uncomfortable last-minute pressure. Those who have found the urgency of a fast-approaching deadline conducive to productivity (and even best work) may need to modify their approach slightly in the face of competing demands.

PLACE

As well as managing your time, it is also advisable to consider your place of study. Different study activities will fit varying circumstances. Some gentle reading may be easily accommodated at home even with background noise, whilst structuring your first written piece of work will likely call for quieter surroundings. Many hospital Trusts have libraries which offer uninterrupted space and digital resources. Of course, university libraries provide comprehensive services and learning development teams who can support students in acquiring a range of study skills.

Working at home has its advantages. If you have an identified space with a desk and good lighting where you can study undisturbed, this may be the best arrangement. Kitchen tables may only be able to function as desks for a few weeks; after this, packing and unpacking piles of books and papers becomes frustrating and time-consuming and can even lead to the loss of a precious set of notes.

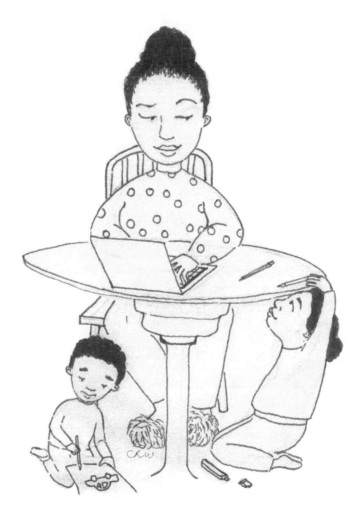

ILLUSTRATION NO. 7.1B   Young mum studying on laptop.

PERSONAL LEARNING STYLES

It is generally agreed that individuals learn in different ways, but it may be some time since you have last tested out your own learning preferences. Return to Practice courses are usually quite short and therefore touching base with the approach that works best for you can save time and effort.

There are many tools designed to help us identify our preferred learning style. We recommend the Learning Styles Questionnaire (Honey and Mumford 1986) because it provides insight into how we learn in practice as well through study. We have included a format here adapted from the NHS Leadership Academy (2018); however, there are many other versions readily accessible online. Scores are distributed across four distinct learning modes and have been helpfully summarised by Common and Maslin-Prothero (2011).

	Learning Styles Questionnaire This questionnaire will help to identify your learning preferences. Tick the statements you agree with. There are no right or wrong answers.	
1	I often take reasonable risks if they're justified.	
2	I tend to solve problems using a step-by-step approach, avoiding any 'flights-of-fancy'.	
3	I have a reputation for having a no-nonsense style.	
4	I often find that actions based on 'gut feel' are as sound as those based on careful thought and analysis.	
5	What matters most is whether something works in practice.	
6	When I hear about a new idea or approach, I immediately start working out how to apply it in practice.	
7	I am keen on self-discipline such as watching my diet, taking regular exercise and sticking to clear routines.	
8	I take pride in doing a thorough job.	
9	I get on best with logical, analytical people and less well with spontaneous, 'irrational' people.	
10	I take care over the interpretation of data available to me and avoid jumping to conclusions.	
11	I like to reach a decision carefully after weighing up many alternatives.	
12	I'm attracted more to novel, unusual ideas than to practical ones.	
13	I don't like 'loose ends' and prefer to fit things into a coherent pattern.	
14	I like to relate my actions to a general principle.	
15	In discussions I like to get straight to the point.	
16	I prefer to have as many sources of information as possible – the more data to mull over the better.	
17	People who don't take things seriously enough usually irritate me.	
18	I prefer to respond to events on a spontaneous, flexible basis, rather than planning things out.	

19	It worries me if I have to rush a piece of work to meet a tight deadline.	
20	I tend to judge people's ideas on their practical merits.	
21	I often get irritated by people who want to rush into things.	
22	It is more important to enjoy the present moment than to think about the past or future.	
23	I think that decisions based on a thorough analysis of all the information are sounder than those based on intuition.	
24	I enjoy contributing ideas just as they occur to me.	
25	On balance I talk more than I listen.	
26	In discussion I get impatient when people lose sight of the objective.	
27	I enjoy being the one that talks a lot.	
28	In discussions I often find that I am the realist, keeping people to the point and avoiding 'cloud nine' speculations.	
29	I like to ponder many alternatives before making up my mind.	
30	In discussions with people I often find I am the most dispassionate and objective.	
31	In discussions I'm more likely to adopt a 'low profile' than to take the lead and do most of the talking.	
32	On balance I do the listening rather than the talking.	
33	Most times I believe the end justifies the means.	
34	Group objectives and targets should take precedence over individual feelings and objections.	
35	I do whatever is needed to get the job done.	
36	I quickly get bored with methodical, detailed work.	
37	I am keen on exploring basic assumptions, principles and underpinning theories underpinning things and events.	
38	I like meetings to be run on methodical lines, sticking to a laid down agenda.	
39	I steer clear of subjective or ambiguous topics.	
40	I enjoy the drama and excitement of a crisis situation.	

Record where you placed the ticks on the questionnaire

1	4	12	18	22	24	25	27	36	40	Activist	
8	10	11	16	19	21	23	29	31	32	Reflector	
2	7	9	13	14	17	30	37	38	39	Theorist	
3	5	6	15	20	26	28	33	34	35	Pragmatist	

(continued)

(continued)

Summary
The activist
- Enjoys new experiences and challenges
- Enjoys an environment of changing activities
- Likes being the centre of attention
- Appreciates the chance to develop ideas through interaction and discussion with others

The activist thrives and develops in an environment that utilises some of the following teaching and learning strategies: group work, seminars, discussions, debates and workshops.

The reflector
- Appreciates the opportunity to reflect prior to making a decision or choice
- Prefers to listen and observe others debating and discussing issues
- Would choose to work independently of others

The reflector is someone who prefers to work on his or her own, through individual study and project work. Reflectors are likely to prefer lectures.

The pragmatist
- Likes linking theory with practice
- Enjoys problem solving
- Appreciates the opportunity to develop practical skills

The pragmatist will enjoy those learning experiences that involve problem-solving activities, practical sessions, clinical experiences and work-based projects.

The theorist
- Enjoys theories and models
- Thrives on problem solving which involves understanding and making sense of complex issues
- Likes structure and making the link to theories

The theorist will benefit and enjoy those sessions that use problem solving, evaluating material and discussing theories with colleagues and teachers.
Common and Maslin-Prothero (2011)

Source: Adapted from Honey & Mumford (1986).

Most of us will arrive with results across all four areas but will discover a propensity perhaps in one or two. As authors, we find ourselves to be predominantly a mix of pragmatist and reflector!

Another system operates by understanding how each of us processes learning through our five senses. The VAK system was devised to reveal individual learning preferences, often resulting in confirming something that perhaps we have always known intuitively (Fleming 2006). VAK stands for – Visual, Auditory and Kinaesthetic. In some versions, a Read/Write dimension has been added, turning the acronym into VARK. The system works through interpreting answers to questions in a similar way to Honey and Mumford's approach. The strength of the exercise lies in how each person takes their findings to inform future learning. We have presented here a sample of some of the VAK questions with an accompanying summary. This will give you a flavour of what is involved; however, for a more accurate result, we would recommend that you locate the full questionnaire online. We have included a link in the reference list at the end of the chapter.

VAK Learning Styles Self-Assessment Questionnaire

Please note the answer that most represents how you generally behave.

1. When I operate new equipment I generally:
   (a) read the instructions first
   (b) listen to an explanation from someone who has used it before
   (c) go ahead and have a go, I can figure it out as I use it

2. When I need directions for traveling I usually:
   (a) look at a map
   (b) ask for spoken directions
   (c) follow my nose and maybe use a compass

3. When I cook a new dish, I like to:
   (a) follow a written recipe
   (b) call a friend for an explanation
   (c) follow my instincts, testing as I cook

4. When I am choosing a holiday I usually:
   (a) read lots of brochures
   (b) listen to recommendations from friends
   (c) imagine what it would be like to be there

5. When I am learning a new skill, I am most comfortable:
   (a) watching what the teacher is doing
   (b) talking through with the teacher exactly what I am supposed to do
   (c) give it a try myself and work it out as I go

6. If I am choosing food off a menu, I tend to:
   (a) imagine what the food will look like
   (b) talk through the options in my head or with my partner
   (c) imagine what the food will taste like

7. When I listen to a band, I can't help:
   (a) watching the band members and other people in the audience
   (b) listening to the lyrics and the beats
   (c) moving in time with the music

8. I choose household furnishing because I like:
   (a) their colours and how they look
   (b) the descriptions the salespeople give me
   (c) the textures and what it feels like to touch them

9. When I am anxious, I:
   (a) visualize the worst-case scenarios
   (b) talk over in my head what worries me most
   (c) can't sit still, fiddle and move around constantly

10. I feel especially connected to other people because of:
    (a) how they look
    (b) what they say to me
    (c) how they make me feel

11. When I have to revise for an exam, I generally:
    (a) write lots of revision notes and diagrams
    (b) talk over my notes, alone or with other people
    (c) imagine making the movement or creating the formula

(continued)

(continued)

12. If I am explaining to someone I tend to:
    (a) show them what I mean
    (b) explain to them in different ways until they understand
    (c) encourage them to try and talk them through my ideas as they do it

13. I really love:
    (a) watching films, photography, looking at art or people watching
    (b) listening to music, the radio or talking to friends
    (c) taking part in sporting activities, eating fine foods and wines and dancing

14. Most of my free time is spent:
    (a) watching television
    (b) talking to friends
    (c) doing a physical activity or making things

15. I first notice how people:
    (a) look and dress
    (b) sound and speak
    (c) stand and move

16. If I am angry, I tend to:
    (a) keep replaying in my mind what it is that has upset me
    (b) raise my voice and tell people how I feel
    (c) stamp about, slam doors and physically demonstrate my anger

17. I find it easiest to remember:
    (a) faces
    (b) names
    (c) things I have done

18. I remember things best by:
    (a) writing notes or keeping printed details
    (b) saying them aloud or repeating words and key points in my head
    (c) doing or practicing the activity or imagining it being done

19. If I have to complain about faulty goods, I am most comfortable:
    (a) writing a letter
    (b) complaining over the phone
    (c) taking them back to the store or posting them back to head office

20. I tend to say:
    (a) I see what you mean
    (b) I hear what you are saying
    (c) I know how you feel

Now add up how many As, Bs and Cs you selected

Visual learning style (Mostly As)
Someone with a visual learning style prefers to see or observe things, including pictures, diagrams, demonstrations, displays, handouts, films, flipchart, etc. Phrases such as 'Show me' or 'Let's have a look at that' will be used. Individuals with this learning style like to work from lists and are best able to perform a new task after reading the instructions or watching someone else do it first.

(continued)

Auditory learning style (Mostly Bs)

Auditory learners prefer the transfer of information through listening to the spoken word, or to sounds and noises. These people will use phrases such as 'Tell me' or 'Let's talk it over' and like to perform a new task after listening to instructions from an expert. Individuals with this learning style are happy being given spoken instructions and can remember song lyrics they hear!

Kinaesthetic learning style (Mostly Cs)

This learning style shows a preference for physical experience – touching, feeling, holding, doing. There will be a tendency for phrases such as 'Let me try' or 'How do you feel?' Individuals with a kinaesthetic learning style will be best able to perform a new task by trying it out, learning as they go. These are the people who like to experiment and prefer not to look at the instructions first!

People usually have a blend of all three learning styles with one predominating. Some have a very strong preference whilst others will show a more even mixture of two, or less commonly, three styles. There is no right or wrong learning style. The key message is that knowing your preferences will help direct you towards methods of learning which are likely to suit you best.

UNDERSTANDING COURSE REQUIREMENTS

University courses are structured into modules which carry credits. The modules that make up three-year undergraduate programmes eventually award successful students with the number of credits (usually three hundred and sixty) required to achieve their degree. Return to Practice courses are shorter and often part time, usually consisting of one or two modules, ranging between twenty and thirty credits. Most, but not all, are set at Level 6 which matches the third year of an undergraduate nursing programme.

Educational levels of attainment are determined by government bodies and presented in descriptors which can be challenging to interpret. Level 6 equates to degree qualification and aligns with a range of key qualities and skills including the ability to solve problems and make sound judgements. Students at this level should have a systematic understanding of their field of study and be able to engage in critical commentary and evaluation of current research. An appreciation of the provisional nature of knowledge should be demonstrated along with the ability to identify and challenge assumptions and make decisions in unpredictable contexts. Transferable skills include the exercise of initiative and personal responsibility (Quality Assurance Agency for Higher Education (QAA) 2014). Whilst all of this may sound formal and weighty, we will go on in this chapter to unpack and demystify some of these elements. Courses are designed to embed the knowledge and skills needed for successful achievement at the required academic level. Each module has its own written specification which includes information about entry requirements, course content, assessment and learning outcomes.

As with all occupations and professions, higher education has its own terminology. Module specifications provide a good example of the use of educational wording which for the uninitiated, can be baffling. In many ways, this does not affect students because course information is also decoded and conveyed by course teams.

LEARNING OUTCOMES

What is a learning outcome? In simple terms, learning outcomes tell the student what they will need to demonstrate to pass the module. Unfortunately, such statements can be written in a compressed and unfamiliar language which can present barriers to understanding. Words such as 'analyse', 'critically evaluate' and 'apply knowledge of' are commonly used and have precise meanings, pointing to and reflecting nuanced levels of academic attainment. It is therefore essential that course teams explain these terms so that students are aware of what is expected of them. Where this is not forthcoming, for whatever reason, we would urge students to question, seeking clarity wherever the language seems inaccessible.

A FRAMEWORK FOR ACADEMIC WRITING

Educational terminology in higher education is not limited to module specifications. It can also be found in module handbooks, guidelines for assessment, descriptors concerning academic grading and marking comments. The central tenets of academic writing hinge on some of these key terms with one well-known framework offering some clarity. Bloom's Taxonomy (Anderson and Krathwohl 2000) is a long-established and enduring model for classifying thinking and writing skills. It sets out a hierarchy of levels, starting with the lowest and simplest form of academic activity and progressing up to higher and more complex areas. Originally intended as a tool for categorising educational goals, or learning outcomes, Bloom's Taxonomy (see Figure 7.2)

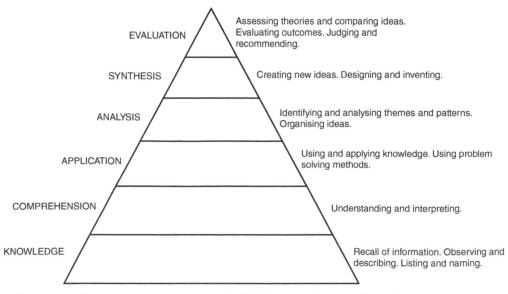

FIGURE 7.2   Blooms taxonomy. *Source:* Modified from Anderson and Krathwohl 2000.

persists as an underlying theoretical root for marking criteria and is still used in many University courses.

Using this framework and the interpretations provided, we can now see that 'analysing' is concerned with identifying patterns or themes and is set at quite a high level. 'Application' is lower down the triangle and is used to problem solve, taking knowledge from one context to another. At the highest level is 'evaluation' where judgement is needed to weigh one idea against another. This then begins to throw some light on what a learning outcome might mean when it asks students to 'critically evaluate' or 'apply knowledge'.

Whilst still acknowledging that there is progression from remembering and understanding facts to being able to contrast and appraise them, revised versions of Bloom's work seek to downplay the hierarchical dimension, preferring instead to highlight how each component relies and builds on the others (Anderson and Krathwohl 2000). This is worth noting and a reminder that whilst models provide structure and guidance, the reality is often a more interrelated picture. In this spirit and mindful that most returners will have memories of studying previously, we have endeavoured here to align the framework more broadly, recognising where each element can be applied to the Return to Practice journey.

Knowledge

During your first few weeks it is likely that knowing or retrieving facts and information will feel of utmost importance. You will need to build your knowledge, acquainting yourself with current thinking, assimilating different processes and learning new skills. In your academic writing, you will need to reference your work, drawing on reputable contemporary published sources to support statements of fact. Once a basis of new understanding feels secure, you are then able to move on to challenge and question. The message, therefore, is that whilst level 6 nurse students need to demonstrate critical thinking, they cannot do this until they have first updated the knowledge, or *evidence base*, for their practice.

Comprehension

This level marks the way in which knowledge is interpreted. In academic terms, it relates to your ability to demonstrate understanding of the literature by being able to paraphrase what you have read. It is nearly always better to use your own words rather than directly quoting others because this shows comprehension and an ability to recast facts and ideas into your own words.

Application

The ability to apply knowledge from one place to another is vital. Published information is often framed within a context; however, to make sense of individual practice situations, healthcare practitioners need to draw on and connect different areas of understanding.

The example below shows how a returning nurse was able to use her understanding of non-verbal communication to compensate for the barriers created by her face mask.

Returner's Excerpt

The use of face masks due to COVID-19 has impacted communication. They create a physical barrier to effective communication by impeding speech intelligibility and limiting rapport building and the picking up of non-verbal cues (Marler et al. 2021). Therefore, it was important when speaking to my patient that I emphasised non-verbal communication such as expression with eyes and hands, body movements and posture. I also talked more slowly but not more loudly due to confidentiality issues (Mheidly et al. 2020; Marler et al. 2021).

You will be able to show your application of theory to practice both in your conversations with assessors and supervisors, and through using information from a range of published sources to support the points you want to make.

Analysis

Once the knowledge base feels more familiar and you can apply your reading to your practice, you will be able to start to question. Being able to put forward an argument to justify a stance or support a view is crucial to professional working (Maslin-Prothero 2011). A questioning approach signifies movement from the descriptive to the analytical. In your written work, you will be critiquing the literature and sequencing ideas into logical discussion. This is about looking beneath the surface to perceive underlying themes. It is important to engage with and balance a range of viewpoints, closely referencing and contrasting and comparing different authors. In her excellent chapter on critical thinking, Cottrell (2019) reminds us that, left undisciplined, our brains tend to race for quick and easy answers, often running along old established tracks where unconscious bias and subjective ideas take the lead. For example, the wearing of a head covering could be due to religious observance, but it could also be because your patient is suffering from alopecia. Critical thinking means being on the alert, prepared to regularly challenge first impressions so that we can develop greater awareness of our own assumptions and shortcut thinking. It also means not taking for granted the reasoning of others but asking questions to obtain clarity. When we scrutinise the spoken or written word in depth, we are more likely to understand the precise detail of an argument and we can then reach a more open-minded and objective stance.

Synthesis

Having broken things down into parts and examined individual elements, synthesis puts everything back together to form a new whole. Perhaps receiving less focus than analysis, synthesising is a creative activity which concentrates on seeing things afresh and looking for new solutions. You may have an opportunity to initiate change in your practice placement. After some weeks in a theatre setting, observing new students at a loss when asked to fetch surgical equipment and himself struggling to find instrument packs in the store cupboard, one returner took steps to initiate a more logical system, re-organising what went where on the shelves. His reading told him that efficient storage saved time and reduced stress especially in hospital theatres (NHS Institute for Innovation and Improvement 2020). With this underpinning evidence he was able to make an argument to support his proposed change (Maslin-Prothero 2011). It transpired that many staff had experienced similar difficulties, and his actions were met with praise all round.

Evaluation

Finally, evaluation is about weighing the evidence and assessing significance. There will come a point in your return to practice journey where prior experience will start to merge and fuse with new insights and understandings, enabling you to gauge your own professional development and make judgements on issues such as quality and clinical effectiveness. We recall one student returning to community nursing who spotted an aspect of unsafe practice in the way oxygen cylinders were being stored at a patient's home. She was able to quickly assess the situation and alert the relevant team so that a safer solution could be put in place.

KNOWLEDGE FOR PRACTICE: THE EVIDENCE BASE

The academic components of RTP courses come in all shapes and sizes – essays, reflective accounts, care studies – to name a few. Some courses focus considerable attention on written assignments, whilst others ask for very little, choosing instead to place most weight on practice assessments. Whatever the format, however, you will need to demonstrate an understanding of the evidence base which underpins your practice.

Knowledge within the healthcare professions is drawn from a range of disciplines including human biology, medicine, social science, pathophysiology and psychology. This is especially true for nursing and midwifery where practice is grounded in a rich diversity of understandings. This supporting knowledge provides the evidence base for what we do and can be divided into many kinds of categories. We can see it as subject areas such as pharmacology and communication skills; it can be viewed in broad practice areas or nursing fields such as accident and emergency, rehabilitation, learning disabilities or mental health. In addition, the literature charts an evolving picture as to what this evidence base should be, reflecting a movement towards a more inclusive perspective which recognises that alongside primary research, must also be the voices of patients (service users) and carers describing their experiences and informing us with their responses to the care we give (Davies and Gray 2017).

The following excerpt is taken from a published collection of stories written by service users (Allen and Lilley 2009). The book shares how it feels to be on the receiving end of care. Here an Occupational Therapist is hospitalised after sustaining a serious fall. This reflection speaks of what she comes to know as a patient going through rehabilitation.

A Service User's Perspective

After three days of lying flat I was to get up and go to the bathroom. I asked for a wheelchair because I was concerned I would be light-headed after lying flat for so long, but the policy was that I should walk. I think I managed about three steps before I fainted and was very angry that no one had considered I knew myself well enough to know what might happen.

    The physio was a joy. Maybe because I saw him as a colleague, but I think because he treated me as an individual, I felt we could work through things together... He listened to my woes and anxieties and took notes. He went to get my x-rays and showed them to me (something no one else had felt they should do despite my requests) and we talked through what my rehabilitation was likely to look like....

    ...Learning to go up and down stairs in the physio gym (the criteria it seems for discharge) caused me far more concern than I could have imagined. My fear of falling again was in overdrive, never have four steps seemed so high, but 'doing stairs' was the test to pass, so up and down I went on wobbly, painful legs, determined to pass muster. I had never realised how anxious people could become at such a seemingly small exercise, nor how much power conducting such a 'test' gives to a therapist, nor how small a patient's world becomes, and how quickly.

This insight into a service user's perspective confronts healthcare workers with some difficult truths. As an experienced practitioner, she is used to communicating her knowledge and having it respected. In this situation, however, she has lost this authority and the knowledge she does tries to voice about herself is only listened to by one other person. When it comes to the stairs assessment – something which as a therapist she has conducted for many patients – she is shocked to discover how stressful this experience turns out to be. Her eventual hope is that this new understanding will help her to support future patients with greater empathy. In such a way, practitioners infuse their formal subject-based knowledge with their own experiential learning providing each with a working evidence base for practice unique to them. In the previous chapter we explored this kind of practice knowing, generated mostly through individual reflection (Higgs and Titchen 2001; Rolfe 2011).

    The nature of nursing knowledge is continually changing in response to new research and the needs of patients. It may be relevant and appropriate for its time, but it must also be subject to constant scrutiny and updating. Graduate study draws on the facts and thinking set out in current academic literature but must also embrace a spirit of inquiry generated from the stance that all knowledge is provisional (McMillan 2021). Our professional development hinges on asking questions and challenging the status quo when it does not align with the realities of practice. In the following written extract, a returning student is faced with an uncertain practice dilemma which causes her to examine and weigh up the existing evidence base. Mr. X has been upset by an episode of diarrhoea overnight which has contaminated his pressure ulcer dressing.

Returner's Account

I was concerned about the integrity of the dressing, and that the wound may be at risk of infection if contaminated by faeces. Faeces can damage the skin and lead to issues such as Incontinence-Associated Dermatitis (IAD) and Moisture Associated Skin Damage (MASD). Moisture on the skin greatly increases the risk of pressure ulcers (Fletcher 2020; Beckman et al. 2020; NICE 2014) and, of course, wound infections can impact the healing process and potentially lead to sepsis (Sepsis Alliance 2019). This would suggest that faecal incontinence presents a serious risk to skin integrity, healing of wounds and can ultimately be detrimental to patient health. The dressing was not due to be changed until later that afternoon: however, I made an evidence-based decision to inspect the wound before then. I needed to think through any potential disadvantages to carrying out the dressing change earlier than planned; these could include risking untimely exposure of the wound with potential for bacterial contamination and disturbing any healing tissue (National Pressure Ulcer Advisory Panel (NPUAP) 2016). I also wanted to consider Mr. X's psychological needs as he was not prepared for the wound dressing to be changed until later that day. I needed to involve Mr. X in any decisions about his care as promotes a sense of ownership and autonomy (Coultier & Collins 2011). I discussed my concerns with Mr. X and he consented for me to assess the area (NMC 2018). Guided by the evidence on pressure ulcer pain management (NPUAP 2016) I reassured Mr. X that he would be made as comfortable as possible by co-ordinating his pain medication with the procedure. Mr. X agreed to the plan and on inspection it was evident that the dressing did need to be changed.

The NMC clearly state that it is important to recognise the limits of your competence, and this is particularly important working within the role of a student nurse (NMC 2018). In compliance with the NMC Code, I discussed the situation with my supervisor. Although evidence-based guidelines discourage too frequent dressing changes, they do not make provision for an individual deviation from the usual plan of care. Clinical guidelines and care plans aim to support clinicians in the decision-making process by standardising care and encouraging best practice (McLachlan et al. 2020). Tools such as decision trees, flow charts and algorithms use step-by-step procedures with evidence suggesting that these methods enable higher levels of safety in controlling risks in patient health (Standing 2017). However, the tools rely on an outcome being predictable and this experience demonstrates that not all scenarios can be pre-determined, suggesting the tools can be somewhat limited (Engebretsen et al. 2016). Appraising clinical judgements provides an opportunity to identify knowledge and skills deficits enabling adjustments to be made to practice (Jasper et al. 2013).

We see that the returner has arrived at a place of uncertainty having established that the situation seems to draw on conflicting areas of knowledge. The clinical guidelines for pressure ulcer management offer a standardised response which here must be questioned. Her search for the best course of action for her patient leads to a comparing and contrasting of evidence bases and her judgement enables her to find the right solution. Policies and clinical guidelines are informed by primary research findings and are essential to evidence-based practice because they provide practitioners with a current and reliable working knowledge. They are standardised to ensure consistently wide application (National Institute for Health and Care Excellence (NICE) 2018). However, everyday practice is often an unpredictable or 'swampy lowland' requiring us to look beneath the surface to pinpoint knowledge specific and precise enough to apply to each patient encounter (Schon 1987). Returning students are well-positioned to combine past reserves of nursing experience with fresh insights afforded through the updating of knowledge.

READING

Studying starts with reading. One of the most accessible and well-known writers on study skills refers to the 'centrality of reading' in higher education (Cottrell 2019). Her tips for effective reading are wide-ranging and well worth noting.

In daily life we engage with reading tasks at varying levels. For instance, the skills we use to glean information from road signs differs markedly from those needed to follow the instructions for flatpack furniture. A quick scan accomplishes the first task; the second requires a methodical step-by-step approach (and often much patience!). Part of your return to practice updating will necessitate the reading of research articles which will demand yet another level of skills: only careful, in-depth involvement with the text will enable a full understanding and appraising of what is being discussed. Initially, though, a selective approach which concentrates on the abstract or introduction and the final recommendations, may be all that is needed to judge how useful the article may be. Martindale (2011) encourages us to engage in active reading, adopting the best reading strategy for the task in hand. Cottrell agrees, encouraging us to cultivate an expert 'reader voice' (Cottrell 2019, p. 220). Using an internal running commentary as we read helps to develop a questioning approach, drawing us in to engage critically with the subject matter and appraise its quality. Remember also to factor in your best time and place for reading, and work with your personal learning tendencies: audio learners, for example, may prefer to read aloud and then listen to the recordings.

Whilst acknowledging that reading takes time, many students enthuse about reconnecting with their professional knowledge base as they look back on their return journey. They advise on the importance of reading widely and following lines of inquiry raised through practice. Some express a sense of empowerment and excitement for future study.

Words of Wisdom

Studying makes you read around topics and gives you confidence because your knowledge increases.
Make sure you allow time to read and research before writing.
Reading changes your perspective. It motivates you towards professional development.
You will need more time than you think for researching around subjects.
I really enjoyed reading and studying – it's so interesting.

LIBRARIES

University libraries are large friendly places, open for long hours and often purpose-built to accommodate quiet study areas and lively group work. Facilities include computer and Wi-Fi access, photocopiers and printers and comfortable seating with a café usually never far away! Most texts are still available in hard copy and book borrowing time periods are usually generous. As you would expect, many resources are now available in digital format and advice on how to access this information is always on hand to guide both students and staff. Library teams embrace specialisms across subject disciplines so there will be a Faculty or Subject librarian with expertise concerning healthcare and nursing sources; often course inductions will include a library session run by these members of staff. Many returners feel overwhelmed at the prospect of searching the literature using digital systems, so we asked our academic librarian for some guidance. Her helpful advice has been captured in the following sections.

Literature Searching

When we think about literature searching it can feel like a foreign concept, but you have many of the skills already. They are the same that you have used to compare prices for a washing machine or car insurance. However, whilst it is tempting to jump straight into a book or journal, looking for relevant material, it is important to follow a logical process which includes planning and evaluating what you find.

Planning

Think about what words link to your topic or the experience about which you are reflecting. Remember that search engines and databases do not read – they literally search for the words you input. Therefore, keep focused on keywords, and the simpler, the better. There are also lots of different ways to describe things, so try to think about any other keywords you could use. A good strategy is to consider the medical terminology, layman's terms and any abbreviations or acronyms you might use in practice. Write these words down to use in your search. For example, if you want information about infection control, you might look at search terms like hand washing, aseptic technique and hygiene. A good idea is to imagine that you are explaining the topic to someone who does not know anything about it, making a note of the words you use. If you are unfamiliar with the subject matter, start with a textbook from your reading list. Your tutors will have put together a list of useful resources (books, journal articles, videos, websites). Some of these will provide a good introduction to the topic; if you refer to the table of contents or index page you will be able to see what information is contained. These notes and keywords will be the basis of your search.

Searching

What type of information do you need? Information related to practice may be first sought from clinical policies and guidelines accessed via the internet, government websites and the wider web. These sources can complement the literature you find in your textbooks or journal articles. Unfortunately, not everything is available in the same place. You will have to search your library catalogue or discovery service, databases and the internet, so give yourself time.

Databases are a great place to search for subject-specific information. It can take a while to feel comfortable searching them, but there may be some useful library help guides or videos that can guide you. Use your keywords and begin by searching broadly. Start with the main concept or topic and then slowly add additional keywords to help focus and refine your search. An example of a topic might be 'infection control' – you can narrow this down by looking for 'infection control' AND 'community'. Using AND to add additional keywords related to your topic helps to refine your search. If you want to expand your results perhaps by looking at a large geographical area, you can add a 'search string' using the name of the country: for example, 'UK OR United Kingdom OR England OR Wales OR Northern Ireland OR Scotland OR Great Britain OR GB'. The use of OR keeps the search wide – it is an instruction to the search engine or database that you are happy for your results to include any of these words.

Evaluating

As you search for suitable published sources you will need to appraise the quality of what you are reading. Asking questions is a good way to be more critical and less descriptive in your work. The following questions might be helpful:

- **Who** has produced the information? Is it an academic or a practising nurse? Who are they writing for? Who is the intended audience?
- **What** are they saying?
- **Where** is the information from? Is it reliable?
- **When** was it created? Is it up to date?
- **How** did they do it? If it is research, what did they do?

- **Where and what is their evidence?** A good academic source should have clear evidence (normally in the form of references) indicating that what they have read has influenced and helped them to develop their argument.

Words of Wisdom from an Academic Librarian

You have many skills already. Remember to focus on the quality of the information, making sure that it is academic. Take time to think about what you want first, then you can target your search and use your time more effectively.

Feel free to ask for assistance. Library staff are friendly and helpful – they want you to be able to access the resources you need. Remember, it is just a conversation and if they cannot help you, they will always try and find out who can. Library workshops are helpful in giving tips about where to locate what you need more effectively.

Investing time in finding, reading and evaluating the information will help you to write good academic work and the evidence will help you grow in your professional practice.

Here are a few more tips to help you make the most of library services:

- Use the online facilities. University libraries have web pages where you can access services and contact staff.
- For a quick guide, consider going on a library tour – face-to-face or virtual.
- Be careful with photocopying. Don't just collect information – it can create a false sense of security and become expensive.
- If you live some distance from the university, you may find that your local hospital trust library best answers your needs. Talk to your University about inter-library loan access, visit the trust library to see what services are in place or contact your placement provider to explore what might be available.
- There are benefits of spending a full day in the library. Even if this involves a few hours of travel, a purposeful day of quiet study with resources on hand can be very worthwhile. Planning is the key, though – to avoid distractions and prevarication, go with a task and finish approach!

REFERENCING

Why Do We Reference?

We have seen how nursing knowledge is generated from a wide range of sources. Through published writings this knowledge is communicated, disseminated and challenged. Reputable academic outputs are peer reviewed to ensure quality and rigour. As lifelong professional learners we draw on this ever unfolding and progressing evidence base to ensure that our practice remains contemporary and accountable.

When entering a period of formal education, such as a Return to Practice course, you may be required to demonstrate your understanding of that evidence base by using it to support your written work.

First and foremost, the act of referencing pays respect to the authority of published work. The word 'author' comes from 'authority' and is derived from the Latin 'auctoritas' which translates to 'originator'. When we reference, we are acknowledging the origin or author of the ideas being discussed, so it is important to carry out this activity as accurately as we can. Referencing can fill people with dread, but it is an important skill. When we provide a list of the academic sources that have supported our writing, we are also communicating factual details to others. An accurate reference will provide readers with the information they need to find the author, either to verify what you have written or to further their own knowledge. Incorrect referencing is like putting only half the postal address on an envelope; but we will move on to referencing technique in a moment.

Referencing also shows a depth and breadth of reading. If our arguments are underpinned with a range of relevant academic sources, we are bringing to notice not just what we know but also how well we have prepared.

Finally, and importantly, support from published sources also helps us to build balanced and logical discussion. Reference to a cross-section of authors' views and ideas ensures that we are acquainted with different perspectives and can carefully weigh the arguments.

How Do We Reference?

When acknowledging and using published texts in our written work, good academic practice requires us to follow a set of rules. These rules are presented in various formats through a range of academic referencing styles. Universities will determine the system used, with two of the most popular being Harvard and Vancouver. In nursing courses, the preference (and the one we will focus on) is Harvard referencing, characterised by citing author and date in the main text linked to the listed full reference at the end of the work. By way of contrast, the Vancouver style is a numeric system involving footnotes, itemised sources and intext numbering. It is not possible or indeed necessary here to include mention of all referencing systems; however, what should be observed are the paramount principles of consistency and academic integrity.

Academic Integrity and Plagiarism

Academic integrity is concerned with the fundamental values of honesty, fairness, trust, respect and responsibility (Quality Assurance Agency for Higher Education 2018). It points to a practice that has integrity because it combines creative freedom with acknowledgement of the work of others. Any proven attempt to breach these values constitutes academic misconduct; this is deemed unacceptable behaviour in higher education and often results in students receiving significant penalties. The most obvious manifestation of academic misconduct is plagiarism where evidence shows that a student has copied someone else's work without acknowledgement or reference. In today's academia, most written assessments are submitted via an online platform equipped with software to detect copied material. Therefore, it is relatively easy to spot potential transgressions. Assignments receive a Similarity score indicating the percentage of copied text. This may sound alarming. However, if deliberate plagiarism has not taken place, there is nothing to fear. The software can pick up everything including reference lists, direct quotations and often-repeated terms and phrases; therefore, most assignments will show some percentage of similarity. What is important is that this percentage remains low and reflects a composite of tiny matches that come from a range of different sources. A batch of 1%s from many different places is to be expected and entirely in order. Warning lights come on when an overall 20% similarity shows that this percentage comes from one single source, and that on further scrutiny whole sections of text are highlighted with no reference to the author.

Most higher education courses will run sessions on how to avoid plagiarism and are tolerant of early teething problems when students can inadvertently submit copied text because they have not yet learnt to paraphrase effectively. Sometimes it is possible for online platforms to be set up so that students can submit drafts of work formatively, enabling them to identify potential issues and work on improving their skills in this area.

Consistency

Good referencing technique takes practice. Here is what our returners advise:

> **Words of Wisdom**
>
> Referencing academic writing is challenging.
> Do the referencing as you go along.
> Learn to reference early on – it can't be done last minute.
> List published sources fully as you read them – this will save you time later.

The Harvard system stipulates that academic references must be recorded in brief format in the text and fully listed at the end of the work. The golden rule for all academic writing is that all statements of fact or knowledge must be supported with an appropriate published source. This supporting literature will reflect your reading on the topic and help you to build balanced discussion. There are three distinct ways to incorporate references into your sentences. Look at the examples below taken from a returner's reflective account:

(a) Being able to use silence is an important skill in active listening as it enables you to concentrate on the other person's thoughts rather than your own (Worthen 2018).

(b)   Ali (2018) emphasises the point that it is often appropriate for one person to talk more during a conversation.
(c)   Listening is an active process that requires 'empathy, silence, attention to both verbal and nonverbal communication, and the ability to be nonjudgmental and accepting' (Shipley 2010, p. 125).

In the first example we see that the reference is not needed within the sentence and so it is placed in brackets at the end. The second example leaves just the date in brackets, bringing the author in to form part of the sentence and so lending a little more weight to their perspective. In b) type sentences, a common mistake is to place both date and author in brackets: '(Ali 2018) emphasises ... ' The technical point to make is that any part of a reference that is retained in brackets cannot be considered part of the sentence's meaning. Direct quotations, as shown in c), must appear in speech or quotation marks and the page number included in the bracketed information. You will notice slight variations in technique such as in the use of commas, semi-colons and differences in abbreviations; try to follow your university's referencing guidelines and sustain consistency in your technique as much as possible.

Using the Harvard system, listed sources must be recorded in full and alphabetically. Here are the references from the sentence examples set out as if in a reference list, and you will see that the Shipley reference has been listed as an online source with URL information included:

Ali M (2018) Communication skills 5: effective listening and observation skills. Nursing Times. 114(4) 56–57.

Shipley S (2010) Listening: A concept analysis. Nursing Forum. 42(4) 125–134 Accessed 28.6.21. Available at: https://www.proquest.com/docview/733286174?accountid=128348pq-origsite=primo.

Worthen V (2018) The Power of Silence through Active Listening. Equal Measure.

Consistency, therefore, is also about ensuring that all the sources cited in your writing appear in your reference list and vice versa. This can be a tedious checking task which comes at the end of the academic writing process; however, this level of accuracy is a good indicator that you have mastered the required referencing technique and pay attention to detail. It is surprising how easily last-minute references can be missed from lists, so checking in this way helps to establish good practices.

Practical Tips (McMillan 2021)

Here is a summary of helpful referencing tips:

- Start making a list of useful published sources as you go along. You will then have a store of references which you can go back to when you are completing assignments.

- Software tools such as EndNote and RefMe can be used to help manage your store of references. (If these are new to you, ensure that you factor in enough time to become acquainted with how they work.)
- The library may offer workshops or one-to-one appointments to help you. Make the most of what is on offer – it is there to help you succeed.
- Keep referencing guidelines close at hand so you can refer to them easily and practise the technique often.
- Write these sources out in full. This sounds laborious but will save you time in the long run.
- Allow plenty of time for checking and proof reading.

ASSIGNMENT WRITING PROCESS

Return to Practice courses have a short duration with completion of practice proficiencies and academic assignments happening simultaneously. This creates potential pinch-points which can be difficult for students to navigate. It makes good sense, therefore, to try to illuminate this part of the return journey with some guiding comments about the writing process. From start to finish, the process of completing an assignment is often envisaged in three stages. These are planning, writing and editing. Allocating sufficient time for each of these three stages takes forethought and preparation and should help to avoid the pressure of a last-minute rush! We have set out these stages consecutively, although it would be wrong to suggest that they always proceed in an orderly and linear fashion. Often, you may find yourself back with the literature halfway through the writing stage, looking to expand an argument more fully, or needing to re-write a section identified during editing as requiring further attention.

The first phase can take the most time, but if that time has been used well it can shorten the next part of the process. Planning encompasses a range of different activities including literature searching, reading, taking notes, and making decisions about the focus and structure of your work. Ensure that you have a mind map or list of the key points you want to cover. This will help you to stay on track during the writing period.

The general advice about writing is just to launch in! This is easier for some than others. Recalling what works for you and understanding your own pitfalls will be your best guide. The first sentences can often look a bit rough, and it is tempting to stop and labour over them. However, continually censuring and correcting will slow you down and this can be frustrating. Before you know it, you may find yourself getting side-tracked by other tasks such as cleaning the shower or walking the dog! Introductions can constitute especially difficult starting points, so sometimes it is easier to begin with a more concrete topic from the main body of the assignment. Remember to factor in short breaks as needed and try not to feel overwhelmed by the enormity of the task. Keep your plan and any relevant learning outcomes nearby so that you can check that your discussions align evenly with the requirements and your key points.

Editing and writing are two distinct processes. The brain works differently when editing and the conventional wisdom directs us not to try not to do both simultaneously (McMillan 2021). Inevitably this means that most editing comes at the end when the bulk of written work is done, and energy levels can start to flag. This is unfortunate because a final check through can uncover simple mistakes and omissions which up until that point have gone unnoticed. We recommend strongly that you try to reserve a few days before the submission deadline for these checks and reviews. At some point, of course, you must decide enough is enough, and submit the work!

PLANNING

It is important to think through the key areas of your assignment before engaging in literature searching and reading. This will help you to start with a clear focus which can then be widened or narrowed depending on what you find. Mind maps can be useful for sketching out the broad parameters and giving a sense of scope. They can also help with the ordering of your key points and links to published sources.

Peer-reviewed research articles which demonstrate academic rigour and balanced discussion are clearly good choices, but it will be important to consider a broad range of sources which may also include audit reports, literature reviews and clinical guidelines. Check publication dates to ensure that the content is current. Generally, clinically based sources should not go back further than ten years; however, it is quite acceptable to use theoretical literature (for example nursing models and frameworks) and universally acclaimed seminal work that might be older. Non-academic websites, blogs and opinion pieces are unsuitable because they are often subjective or biased and cannot assure accuracy of information.

Writing an assignment requires us to move information from one place to another. We can transfer and store original published work in a variety of different ways. With so much now online it is easy to bookmark references or copy and paste sections of interest for future reading. Printed copies of selected articles (complying of course with copyright regulations) can have areas of text highlighted. In essence, these actions preserve the source material in its original format and are therefore best focused on capturing key reading for information use only. When published literature is moved for the purposes of informing and contributing to an assignment, there are different considerations to be made. Whilst some students manage to write assignments direct from their reading, this approach is fraught with difficulty. Transferring information in this way can risk plagiarism, placing a heavy reliance on paraphrasing which, even if effective, can become arduous and inconsistent when undertaken 'on the go'. Writing that starts too soon after reading may seem undeveloped or superficial because there has been less time for planning and the processing of ideas. When preparing for assignments and accessing published literature, we recommend a middle step or place where information can sit, pre-selected and already partially transformed in readiness for the writing task ahead. A separate online document can be used to store this material, or you may prefer to make notes from the original source, enabling you to gauge the scope of the task and assure your focus.

Note Taking

Try to think back to when you last prepared for a written assignment. What method did you use to record relevant published facts and ideas ready to incorporate into your own work? Physical note taking is thought to aid memory whether this takes the form of journal entries as a precursor to reflective work or a record of key points to discuss in an academic essay or case study. It is an individual activity, reflecting each person's learning preferences and writing style. Some favour a linear format of phrases and abbreviations whilst others may tend towards more visual representations, choosing bubbles, arrows and symbols. Colour coding can be used to identify themes. The method does not matter provided it is a shorthand which makes sense to you and does not merely replicate what you have read. Note taking in all its shapes and forms (handwritten or digital) comes highly recommended as an active process which engages with the reading matter. As we make notes we start to interpret and understand the text, organising our thoughts and making decisions about which points may be relevant to a forthcoming assignment (Masterson and Lloyd-Jones 2011; Cottrell 2019). Importantly, for this process to align with good academic practice and be worth the time invested, notes should be in our own words paving the way for the paraphrasing required in written assessments, and therefore ensuring that authors' views are accurately represented whilst ensuring that their precise words remain uncopied. A good note taking tip is to link points to page numbers so that you can return quickly to the exact reference in the published source.

WRITING

It is tempting to continue to research, amassing an ever-increasing collection of snippets and viewpoints. However, the inclusion of too much information can crowd your work. Students often come to a halt because they have overloaded a short assignment, losing focus because they have opened too many areas or introduced extraneous detail. Be mindful of your assignment remit, your word count and the points you want to make.

Most written assignments in higher education require a discussion-based approach. The aim is not to relay a narrative of events which describes one action after another, but rather to unpick and analyse a topic through the progression of key points. Some descriptive detail will be necessary to set the context and provide definitions, but this should be kept concise. The emphasis is on the development of an informed and coherent debate which sustains throughout, demonstrating critical lines of inquiry into the relevant literature. The main body of your work will be structured into paragraphs, each of which will contain linking points. These points need to be sequenced so that one leads into the next in a logical flow. The following account shows how a returner has been able to create a balanced discussion with the use of clear signposting indicating movement from one viewpoint to another.

Returner's Account

Kraajivanger (2015) purports that the most common reasons for visiting the Emergency Department (ED) are injuries and musculoskeletal symptoms. Patient B had told me previously that he had not accessed primary health support from the GP before coming into ED. There can be a variance between what patients and ED professionals consider appropriate ED use; physical discomfort can be viewed as unjustifiable (Durand et al. 2012). Patients can though presume that their symptoms are too severe to go to the GP and know of course that ED can provide medical care on demand with radiological and laboratory testing available (Durand et al. 2012; Kraajivanger 2015). Patients such as Patient B who choose to present to ED first could be cared for within general practice support (Kraajivanger 2015). Truter et al. (2021) point out that ED could be an expensive resource for back injury as these patients can manage their self-care and recover quickly.

However, I had been involved with Patient B from the beginning of his admission and had already built a rapport with him. I recognised the situation from his perspective, understanding that his anxiety was linked to his pain and difficulty walking and that these were essential factors in his seeking care in the ED (Coster et al. 2017; Grocott & McSherry 2018). I needed to provide reassurance, communicated through my verbal and non-verbal interactions, demonstrating politeness and courtesy (Hermann et al 2019). Person-centred care requires effective communication to enhance patient psychological and physical outcomes (Lofti et al. 2019; Blackburn et al. 2019).

Remember that an informed understanding of the evidence is not demonstrated by studding your work with repeated direct quotations – all this shows is that you can accurately replicate the written word! Students frequently ask how many references they should include. The answer is not straightforward. Slotting volumes of references into the text may be ineffectual if they just sit there, floating and unexplained. Your discussions need to show that you have explored or engaged with the literature and understand the significance of what you have read (Maslin-Prothero 2011). Consequently, it is better to use fewer references well: often this will reflect both breadth and depth. Judgement is also exercised as to how closely you reference. Each reference must be linked to a statement. A word here on the primary and secondary sources may also be helpful. A primary source is the one you have accessed and read, whilst secondary sources are those referenced within the primary one. Whenever possible, it is best to cite the primary source because this ensures that you are reflecting the original intention of the author. Reference to a secondary source is sometimes unavoidable, but it is important to remember that this material belongs elsewhere. It has been interpreted and customised to fit a different place, and therefore may not tell its full story.

When developing an argument in your work, take care not to make sweeping statements. They may seem to add impact, but the use of absolutes such as 'always' or 'never' incline towards opinion and can exclude the possibility of an opposing argument (Cottrell 2019, p. 303). For instance, the claim that 'nurses always suffer from insomnia' is clearly questionable; however, a more reasonable statement such as 'studies show that nurses tend to sleep less than the rest of the population', followed by a supporting reference, sounds much more credible and reflects the reality of the situation. Our academic discussions must demonstrate an awareness of the provisional nature of knowledge; words such as 'suggest' or 'indicate' make an allowance that things may change and therefore reflect a balanced viewpoint.

Authorities on academic writing agree unanimously that clarity is vital (Masterson & Lloyd-Jones 2011). Cottrell (2019, p. 303) advises against the use of bullet points, explaining that academic writing should be presented as 'continuous prose'. Meaning can be lost or compromised in long winded and elaborate sentences, so take care to aim for succinctness. The use of the first person in reflective work is needed, as we have already seen; however, formal academic work requires a more impersonal approach – 'It has been stated' or 'There is a need to'.

Introductions set the scene, confirm the topic and provide an explanation of what will be covered. They are crucial to most written assignments. Many find it is easier to create these opening statements once the bulk of the main body is in place. The importance of a good conclusion, on the other hand, is often underestimated. A common mistake is to settle for a skimpy last paragraph which merely repeats the introduction in shortened form. Whilst they should not break new ground, conclusions can be dynamic because they pull together and evaluate key findings. They have the power to clarify and elevate a piece of writing.

EDITING

Editing is an essential but often under-estimated activity. It enables us to see afresh something that has become too familiar. Several revisits are recommended because when we re-read work something previously unseen is likely to pop out (McMillan 2021).

A first reading aloud to self and others will pick up any obvious areas that do not make sense. This can be particularly helpful if English is not your first language. We can make assumptions when we turn our thoughts into writing, perhaps failing to provide enough context or not sign posting sufficiently from one sentence to the next. The sequencing of points should be logical with the correct use of connecting words such as 'however' and 'consequently' which serve as signposts directing the reader through your work. When we listen to how our sentences sound often issues come to light. Ears hear what eyes do not always pick up (McMillan 2021). This first reading through will help to check the overall sense and flow of the discussion.

Editing will look closely at the content, focus and structure. Does the assignment meet the assessment requirements and learning outcomes? It is not uncommon for students to either forget about the need to section work into paragraphs, or to separate each point so the text takes on the appearance of listed information. If this is an area that you have struggled with in the past, McMillan (2021) provides a detailed guide on how to shape your text into paragraphs which may be helpful. Most assignments require an introduction and conclusion and so it is important that these align with the main body of the work.

Editing also involves condensing or pruning text, removing unnecessary or repeated words. This is vital to comply with word count requirements (usually a 10% allowance either way), but it also produces something cleaner and sharper, nearly always improving the quality of the writing (McMillan 2021). Many people find this activity challenging perhaps because it involves critiquing and chopping out work that has taken effort to produce. During editing, language use and word choices are checked to ensure that an academic writing style has been followed. Everyday English is full of colloquialisms and idioms which we use almost unknowingly, and this means that they can also filter into our writing. Despite their colourful impact, phrases such as 'in a nutshell' and 'in the heat of the moment' should be replaced with more formal and accurate language, such as 'in summary' and 'suddenly and without thinking'. Be alert for overly conversational language which may seem acceptable on first reading. A sentence such as 'It was really hard to talk to the patient' does not provide sufficiently precise information because the word 'really' is too vague and informal. Similarly, make sure that your work does not contain contractions – words such as 'isn't' and 'won't' are too chatty for academic work.

It is essential to make certain that references have been used consistently to support statements of fact. Some areas of knowledge, such as the subtleties of non-verbal communication, are less obvious, so it is important to go through the text carefully. When in doubt, it is always better to over-reference in academic work. Referencing also needs to be accurate both in terms of technique and ensuring that sources cited in the text are also listed and vice versa. If not already addressed, consistency in font style, text size, the use of subheadings and page numbers are also part of this final review.

Proof reading builds on editing and acts as a final quick check for more minor errors in punctuation, spelling, word choice and abbreviation usage. In addition, tenses should be consistent; this can be tricky especially when narrating events where we can sometimes switch into the present tense as we relive the experience. This may be found in diaries and works well in dramatic fiction but is generally not appropriate in academic work. Try to factor in an extra day between completing and submitting your assignment for one last fresh read through.

PERSONAL TUTORIALS

At some point in the course – usually after the midpoint – it is likely that you will have a personal tutorial. As we have seen from the Johari Window, listening to constructive feedback can enable growth and development. Personal tutorials can mark the moment when everything starts to come together. It is therefore crucial to prepare well beforehand so that you can make the best use of your time.

Tutorials may take place online, face-to-face, via email or phone call. They can be fixed events scheduled into your timetable or negotiated arrangements. If your course allows you flexibility, think carefully about what stage in the writing process a tutorial will afford you most benefit. Some students undertake large proportions of assignments and then contact their tutor to check that they are on the right lines. Others may request an early conversation to establish clarity about assignment guidelines and requirements. Try to work out what is best for you. Your personal learning style may also be a factor here: if you are an auditory learner you may prefer to receive verbal feedback; if you tend to learn visually, it might feel more helpful to read written comments via email.

Whatever the arrangement might be, have questions prepared. This will give you the answers you need to progress your work, and it will also help your tutor to gauge your level of understanding. No question is too small or basic, and often the simplest questions can also uncover areas of ambiguity which need to be addressed with the wider student group. Sharing a section of draft work will enable your tutor to provide responses on both content and writing style. University regulations do not permit tutors to comment on large sections of assignments for obvious reasons; however, providing some text with all its details, ideas and points of reference will enable a fruitful discussion and result in feedback which is likely to be specific and therefore more useful. Personal Tutors are also there to provide pastoral support. Unfortunately, difficult circumstances can arise which may threaten to have an impact on your studies. Whenever possible, it is crucial to share problems with your Personal Tutor and the course team.

Words of Wisdom

Your personal tutor is there to guide you. Ring or email them rather than waste time fretting or second guessing. Act closely on their advice: they are experts at getting students through the course.

ADDITIONAL RESOURCES AND SUPPORT

Universities have a range of measures to support students during their studies. These can be small scale actions such as extending assignment deadlines to more substantial steps which may include facilitating study breaks or implementing mitigating circumstances policy. The most important thing is not to put off seeking support: a minor issue which can be easily resolved in the first month can grow into a much trickier problem if it is left until later in the course.

There are also teams in place to offer extra guidance and assistance. As well as library staff, learning development or study skills tutors can help students with learning differences such as dyslexia to access resources and strategies. Finance and counselling teams are also part of student services and whilst less specific to study, this broader support can ease stress and alleviate external pressures.

ACHIEVEMENT

The return to practice journey is a short one and the learning curve is steep. Academic success, therefore, is to be especially cherished and worthy of congratulations. Commenting on this first foray back into academia, many returning nurses are philosophical, observing that with more time and fewer competing commitments they probably could have produced better work. Some have rightly prioritised achievement of practice proficiency. Nonetheless, most academic assignments pass first time. Where grades are awarded, averages between cohorts are consistent and reflect effort and determination.

Like many things, studying gets better with practice. As markers, we often find that a student's most recent piece of work is their best and, of course, some students do very well. Others may receive a lower grade than expected, and this can be disappointing. However, for Cottrell (2019) it is the feedback that matters most. Many nurses go on to further study, so these early steps back into the academic world can telegraph strengths and areas for future development.

> **Words of Wisdom**
>
> A challenge can be a positive experience!
> I really enjoyed the reading.
> Academic achievement brings personal rewards.
> I had not forgotten everything!
> It's exciting and invigorating, but more challenging this time due to family commitments.
> I found it hard work, but fun.
> It is satisfying when it is all done.
> I am looking forward to further study.

REFERENCES

Allen, S. and Lilley, L. (eds.) (2009). *Look at Me and Smile.* University of Northampton.

Anderson, L.W. and Krathwohl, D.R. (eds.) (2000). *A Taxonomy for Learning, Teaching and Assessing: A Revision of Bloom's Taxonomy of Educational Objectives.* Pearson.

Beckman, D., Fletcher, J., Boyles, A., and Fumarola, S. (2020). Prevention and Management of Moisture Associated Skin Damage (MASD) International best practice recommendations.

Buzan, T. (2018). *Mind Map Mastery*. London: Watkins Publishing.

Blackburn, J. Ousey, K., and Goodwin, E. (2019). Information and communication in the Emergency Department. *International Emergency Nursing* 42: 30–35.

Canning, N. (2010). Playing with heutagogy: exploring strategies to empower mature learners in higher education. *Journal of Further and Higher Education* 34 (1): 59–71.

Chinn, S. (2012). Beliefs, anxiety and avoiding failure in mathematics. *Child Development Research* 2012: Article ID396071.

Coster, J.E., Bradbury, J.K., and Cantrell, A. (2017). Why do people chose emergency and urgent care services? a rapid review utilizing a systemic literature search and narrative synthesis. *Academic Emergency Medicine.* 24 (9): 1137–1149.

Common, L. and Maslin-Prothero, S. (2011). Learning skills and styles. In: *Bailliere's Study Skills for Nurses and Midwives*, 4e (ed. S. Maslin-Prothero). Elsevier Limited.

Cottrell, S. (2019). *The Study Skills Handbook*, 5e. Macmillan Study Skills. Red Globe Press.

Coultier A & Collins A (2011). Making shared decision-making a reality: no decision about me, without me. The Kings Fund.

Davies, K. and Gray, M. (2017). The place of service-user expertise in evidence-based practice. *Journal of Social Work* 17 (91): 3–20.

Durand, A-C. Palazzolo, S. Tanti-Harouin, N. Gerbeaux, P. and Sambuc, R. (2012). Nonurgent patients in emergency departments: rational or irresponsible consumers? Perceptions of professionals and patients. *Biomed Central Research Notes* (5): 1–9.

Engebretsen E. Heggen K. Wieringa S. & Greenhalgh T. (2016). Uncertainty and objectivity in clinical decision making. A clinical case in emergency medicine. Medical Healthcare and Philosophy.

Fleming, N.D. (2006). *Teaching and Learning Styles: VARK Strategies*. Christchurch. https://www.hfe.co.uk/learning-styles-questionnaire (accessed May 31st 2022).

Fletcher, J. (2020). Pressure ulcer education 6: incontinence assessment and care. *Nursing Times* 116 (3): 42–44.

Foster, R.G. and Kreitzman, L. (2017). *Circadian Rhythms: A Very Short Introduction*. Oxford University Press.

Grocott, A. and McSherry, W. (2018). The patient experience: informing practice through identification of meaningful communication from the patient's perspective. *Healthcare* 6 (1): 1–14.

Hermann, R. Long, E. and Trotta, R. (2019). Improving patients' experiences communicating with nurses and providers in the emergency department. *Journal of Emergency Nursing* 45 (5): 523– 530.

Higgs, J. and Titchen, A. (2001). *Professional Practice in Health, Education and the Creative Arts*. Blackwell Science.

Honey, P. and Mumford, A. (1986). *Learning Styles Questionnaire*. Peter Honey Publications Ltd.

Jasper, M., Rosser, M. and Mooney, G. (2013). *Professional Development, Reflection and Decision-Making in Nursing and Health Care*. Advanced Healthcare Practice. 2e. Wiley Blackwell.

Marler, H. and Ditton, A. (2021). 'I'm smiling back at you': exploring the impact of mask wearing on communication in healthcare. *International Journal of Language and Communication Disorders* 56 (1): 205–214.

Kraaijvanger, N., Rijpsma, D., van Leeuwen, H., and Edwards, M. (2015). *International Journal of Emergency Medicine* 8 (1): 1–6.

Lotfi, M., Zamanzadeh, V., Valizadeh, L., and Khajehgoodari, M. (2019). Assessment of nurse-patient communication and patient satisfaction from nursing care. *Nursing Open* 6 (3): 1189–1196.

Martindale, K. (2011). Getting the most from reading and lectures. In: *Bailliere's Study Skills for Nurses and Midwives*, 4e (ed. S. Maslin-Prothero). Elsevier Limited.

Maslin-Prothero, S. (ed.) (2011). *Bailliere's Study Skills for Nurses and Midwives*, 4e. Elsevier Limited.

Masterson, A. and Lloyd-Jones, N. (2011). Writing skills and developing an argument. In: *Bailliere's Study Skills for Nurses and Midwives*, 4e (ed. S. Maslin-Prothero). Elsevier Limited.

McLachlan, S., Kyrimi, E., and Dube, K. (2020). Towards standardisation of evidence-based clinical care process specifications.

McMillan, K. (2021). *The Study Skills Book. Your Essential Guide to University Success*, 4e. Pearson Education Limited.

Mheidly, N., Fares, M.Y., Zalzale, H., and Fares, J. (2020). Effect of face masks on interpersonal communication during the COVID-19 pandemic. *Frontiers in Public Health* (8): 1–7.

National Institute Clinical Excellence (NICE) (2014). Pressure ulcers: prevention and management CG179.

National Institute for Health and Care Excellence (2018). Principles for putting evidence-based guidance into practice. https://www.nice.org.uk/Media/Default/About/what-we-do/Into-practice/Principles-for-putting-evidence-based-guidance-into-practice.pdf.

National Pressure Ulcer Advisory Panel, European Pressure Ulcer Advisory Panel and Pan Pacific Pressure Injury Alliance (2016). Prevention and treatment of Pressure Ulcers: Quick reference guide.

Navarre Cleary, M. (2012). Anxiety and the newly returned adult student. *School for New Learning Faculty Publications*. 5-1-2012. Chicago: DePaul University.

NHS Institute for Innovation and Improvement (2020). The productive operating theatre. Building Teams for Safer Care. Available at: https://www.england.nhs.uk/improvement-hub/publication/the-productive-operating-theatre.

NHS Leadership Academy – north-west (2018). Leadership styles questionnaire. Honey and Mumford. https://www.nwacademy.nhs.uk›resource_files.

NMC (2018). The code. Professional standards of practice and behaviour for nurses, midwives and nursing associates. NMC.

The Quality Assurance Agency for Higher Education (QAA) (2014). UK quality code for higher education. part A: setting and maintaining academic standards. The Frameworks for Higher Education Qualifications of UK Degree-Awarding Bodies.

The Quality Assurance Agency for Higher Education (QAA) (2018). QAA Viewpoint: tackling academic misconduct in higher education.

Truter, P. Edgar, D. Mountain, D. and Bulsara, C. (2021). An emergency department optimized protocol for qualitative research to investigate care seeking by patients with non-urgent conditions. *Nursing Open* 8 (2): 628–635.

Race, P. (2001). Using feedback to help students learn. *The Higher Education Academy*https://phil-race.co.uk/wp-content/uploads/Using_feedback.pdf (accessed June 14th 2022).

Roenneberg, T. (2012). *Internal Time. Chronotypes, Social Jet Lag, and Why You're so Tired.* USA: Dumont Buchverlag.

Rolfe, G. (2011). Knowledge and practice. In: *Critical Reflection in Practice* (G. Rolfe, M. Jasper, and D. Freshwater). Butterworth Heinemann.

Schon, D.A. (1987). *Educating the Reflective Practitioner.* San Francisco: Jossey-Bass.

Sepsis Alliance (2019). Sepsis and pressure ulcers; Infected sores can lead to sepsis. Available at https://www.sepsis.org/news/sepsis-and-pressure-ulcers-infected-sores-can-lead-to-sepsis.

Standing, M. (2017). *Clinical Judgement and Decision making in Nursing for Nursing Students, 3e.* Sage Publications.

CHAPTER 8

Re-Entering the Workforce

CELEBRATING SUCCESS

Each return to practice journey is unique, but nearly all will depend to some measure on the goodwill and involvement of others. Partners, children, friends and neighbours will step in to support along the way, whether this is guiding you through technological challenges, cooking meals or walking the dog. We often say that completing this journey successfully may feel like a shared project where all supporters should also receive an award! At the end of the course, there are often mixed emotions including relief, excitement, joy and maybe some trepidation about the way ahead. However, do pause and take the time to savour what you have achieved. Returning to practice is no mean feat; it is important to acknowledge the challenges, the support and all your hard work. Be proud of how far you have come and celebrate your success!

Words of Wisdom

After a nerve wracking wait the results were in... I had not only passed but passed with flying colours. I could not wait to put on that uniform again and call myself a 'Registered Nurse' once more.

Returning to Nursing Practice: Confidence and Competence, First Edition. Ros Wray and Mary Kitson.
© 2023 John Wiley & Sons Ltd. Published 2023 by John Wiley & Sons Ltd.

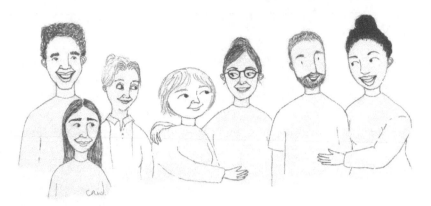

ILLUSTRATION NO. 8.1A   Celebrating success.

THE NMC RE-REGISTRATION PROCESS

Once you have completed the Return to Practice course, the university will advise the NMC of your successful result and make a recommendation for your re-application to the register. You will need to provide two good character references to support your application and your registration fee. The NMC will request a third good health and good character reference from your course leader. Processes will vary from one university to the next, but most will oversee and guide you through this last part of the return journey. Re-entry to the register is a relatively straightforward and mainly administrative procedure. As with many organisations, the NMC now operates using electronic systems, so it is essential to keep your personal details up to date as this will be the point of communication. Each registrant is required simply to create an online account via the NMC website. Registration fees are also paid in this way; this is the principal source of income for the NMC who use the money to support nurse registrants and ensure public protection. Failure to maintain accurate contact details with the NMC is one of the most common reasons for registrations lapsing.

The course aims to leave you feeling ready to return to registered practice, safe and competent to be a nurse again. It cannot prepare you for every situation and you will know that there are still many more things to learn. As you will remember, the transition from student status to registered nurse is exciting but will also bring fresh challenges. Expectations may weigh heavy. It is natural to feel apprehensive about this change in your role and responsibilities. As you have progressed through your placement and grown in confidence and competence, you will have experienced a more reduced level of supervision. Your assessor will have observed and supported you from a distance allowing you to develop and regain your knowledge and skills. You will have acquired experience and proficiencies in leadership, management and decision making, but all under the safety net of supervision. Now you may suddenly feel on your own and this may generate new anxieties.

Words of Wisdom

By the end of the course, I felt exhausted but also thrilled to have completed the course. I was lucky to have a family holiday booked as I finished which gave me a much-needed rest. However, in hindsight I think I put off starting to look for jobs as I was still nervous about becoming a professional nurse again. So, it did take me another couple of months and a phone call from the ward sister encouraging me to apply to the jobs she was going to advertise soon before I felt able to take the leap. Other than the online interview for the RTP course I had not been interviewed for over 11 years, so yet another daunting experience. I am still not sure if interviews are harder or easier online either. During my interview I did explain that I may require a little longer to find my feet because I had been out of nursing for so long. This seemed to be taken on board – I would be classed as a newly qualified nurse, which honestly, made me feel relieved. It was about 5 months after finishing the course before I then started my job. I think this was a bit too long a gap and I feel I would have been suited to going into work again sooner as my confidence had decreased. I had to request for longer supernumerary status, which was thankfully agreed. This really helped me build my confidence, skills, and knowledge again. However due to staff shortages, I found I would be working alongside a bank nurse or agency nurse. This still made me feel under pressure to achieve as other staff often came to me instead of the bank nurse. Thankfully the ward sister made herself available to help me when I needed to ask her advice. It has been a real rollercoaster in the last few months with me feeling like I am achieving and fulfilling my role as a nurse. However, with the demands of some patients and lack of staff at times I have also felt overwhelmed. One area I was not prepared for on returning to work is the pure volume of new starter e-learning that must be completed. This is hours and hours of work with assessments included at the end to check your learning. I have had to use some of my own time for this as it has been so vast. Even with all the challenges returning to the profession that I have had, I am extremely pleased to have become a nurse again, although I have questioned my sanity a few times. I am also wondering if I am better suited to a community nursing role, and I will aim to look for future jobs within this area. My overall advice to anyone considering the Return to Practice course is go for it. It is challenging, but it is worth it.

Whilst delighted to have made the journey, this returner speaks sincerely about her difficult next steps. Any interval between the end of the course and securing employment can allow confidence to wane and insecurities seep in. This can undermine your job search. We can forget what we know as it becomes obscured by what we perceive we are lacking. As this nurse demonstrates, it takes courage and sometimes encouragement from others to press forwards, but it is important to continue the positive trajectory once you have reached the stage of course completion. As we all know, being open and honest about worries or high self-expectations can bring insight and helps enlist the support of others. Remember that returning to a professional role is about confidence and competence so we would urge you to take employment as soon as feasible once you regain your NMC PIN. It may not be your career pathway, but it will allow you to maintain some continuity in the healthcare environment and thus nurture your ongoing growth and development.

Earlier in the book we presented the Code as a source of constancy in directing and advising us especially during challenging times (NMC 2018). In this last chapter it is timely to be reminded of this basis and foundation of our practice. The main objective of the Code is of course public protection and the themes identified are fundamental to this outcome:

- **Prioritise people**
- **Practice effectively**
- **Preserve safety**
- **Promote professionalism and trust**

(NMC 2018)

At its heart is accountability, a familiar concept and guiding star for our everyday practice. We firmly believe that if you hold sight of these informing principles, your nursing actions will be kept safe, supported and effective. In completing your return, you will have achieved the learning outcomes and proved yourself as a safe and competent practitioner. However, the reality is that you have also recommenced a long journey of learning. It is useful to recall Benner and her theories about how we are all progressing from novice to expert (Benner 2001). Nursing as a career has always demanded continuous professional development in various guises and formats, and this will remain ever present as you make the transition from a student back to a registered professional.

CAREER

As you plan your return to registered practice, consider how your circumstances have changed since you last worked as a nurse. Previously you may have thrived on the adrenaline of a fast-paced emergency department where long hours and high pressure were an everyday occurrence. Now, though, you may feel that something more part-time and flexible would suit you better because you have other commitments to juggle, or you just want to spend more time with patients. It could be the reverse: your children have grown up and now you have the freedom to focus more exclusively on your nursing career. Whatever your situation, the maturity and knowing afforded you by life experience may mean that you now look at things differently. These are important considerations. Taking time to think carefully about who you are now and what kind of nursing best fits will help you to set off in the right direction. As we suggested in Chapter 2 a realistic review of your current roles will be helpful along with involving others in your ruminations. Course placements often become the first employment setting for newly returned nurses, and so this may determine how your career starts off again. Nursing is one of the most dynamic and rewarding careers with good prospects for job progression and wide-ranging options in terms of setting, acuity and hours.

Our previous background and experience may also influence our decision as to where we may seek to gain employment or advance our careers. Again, individuals will have different objectives in returning to nursing. It may be part-time work in a less acute area that will gently ease you and perhaps family members back into the reality of a working parent. This will allow everyone to get used to new realities and boundaries and grow in confidence. Alternatively, it may be that you are now keen to grasp opportunities that were not available in your previous time in the profession.

JOB APPLICATIONS

Returnees have often applied and even secured a nursing job before they complete their Return to Practice course. Of course, taking up this post as a registered nurse is conditional on passing the course; however, employers are usually so keen to recruit returners that they will employ them to work in a more junior role prior to re-registration. This works well for all concerned, providing the returner with job security and a comfortable way to acclimatise to new surroundings and colleagues, and enabling the organisation to retain valued staff. Look out for job opportunities and career prospects whilst in placement as often being close to the ground can give you a head start!

In June 2021 there were 38,952 full-time equivalent registered nurses' positions available according to digital data on the NHS website (NHS Digital 2021). However, despite the high number of vacancies, the NHS application process can take from two to six months, so it is a good idea to start applying as soon as possible. All applicants are subject to:

- DBS clearance
- Confirmation of previous employment
- Reference checks
- Pre-employment to ensure you meet the job requirements
- Occupational health checks
- Confirmation the act of registration
- Qualification checks

Most jobs available within the NHS are advertised through NHS jobs and are completed electronically. In addition, Job Fairs and careers events will also provide opportunities for you to see what is out there. You may be aware of and encouraged to apply for vacancies in the clinical setting where you undertake your supervised practice; however, the process will remain the same. The Royal College of Nursing (RCN) has identified four pillars of nursing which you may like to explore once you are ready to look at future career planning and on-going professional development (RCN 2018). They are:

- Clinical practice
- Education
- Leadership
- Research

INTERVIEWS

It may be quite some time since you have undertaken a formal job interview and the prospect may be quite unnerving. However, this is an opportunity to showcase your skills and it is important to prepare. Nurses can struggle to promote themselves, perhaps partly because the skills they possess are difficult to articulate. Consequently, some level of practice or rehearsal will help give a confident performance indicating that you are the best person for the job. Taking the time to think through and note down possible questions and answers will help you to formulate quality responses on the day. Practise these aloud beforehand either with a friend, family member or even alone as voicing your thoughts aloud will reinforce your confidence and ability. As a returner you may feel that you have limited experience in the area you are applying for, so it may be helpful to shadow one of the staff members. An informal chat with a nurse manager will also provide insight. Remember the aim of the interview is to determine if you have the right skills, experience, knowledge, and personality for the role in question. It is important to revisit those transferable skills discussed in earlier chapters as they will demonstrate your strengths in an interview situation.

Feeling nervous is normal and interviewers do take this into consideration. There are simple strategies that can help. Alongside being prepared, having a good understanding of the role and why you think you are the right person will also boost confidence. Be familiar with the job description and refer to the specific skills that are required. It will help to discuss your background and previous experience. It is important to communicate who you are and what you have to offer. Try to be mindful of your non-verbal communication – not easy when you are feeling under pressure! However, try to remember to smile and maintain a good body posture and appropriate eye contact. A firm handshake creates a good impression although, in the brave new world of COVID-19, elbow bumps or a polite nod of the head may be more appropriate! Some deep breathing exercises beforehand may help to allay anxiety. Of course, it is crucial to demonstrate professionalism throughout.

Interviews also offer you the opportunity to determine if the role and organisation is right for you, so do go armed with your own inquiries. What can they offer in terms of preceptorship, clinical supervision, training and development? Although often avoided, the issues of pay grade, benefits and progression need also to be addressed – it is too late once a contract is signed!

BANK NURSING

You may decide to dip your toes before making a commitment to one area or employer and bank nursing offers this opportunity. It allows you to test the water, helping to steer you towards a future area of work. There are various recruitment agencies which will support you in this process. What was previously known as the 'nurse bank' has now become NHS Professionals. This forms the largest pool of both clinical and non-clinical healthcare personnel. Its purpose is to support care settings at times of high demand due to sickness or holiday. Often staff that work in a particular area are recruited via this system. This usually works well as the bank shift will be covered by someone who is familiar with the area, and this in turn reduces stress and facilitates continuity in patient care. It also offers a number of other advantages. The salary is competitive and paid on a weekly basis which is helpful if trying to juggle household budgets. Using an online system, you can pick and choose your shifts according to your availability. Other benefits include access to pension schemes and member-ship support.

This option offers flexibility and good opportunities, but you do need to clearly specify your level of experience and competence. Initially, you may not be prepared to undertake too much responsibility, and, as a returner, you would not be expected to work in areas without support. Clarifying your expectations ensures that you stay within your scope of practice and demonstrates insight and assertiveness. Of course, it is feasible to explore ways of developing your clinical and management skills, so that you could take on additional responsibilities. Nursing staff are a valued resource within healthcare organisations so it vital that recruited staff are retained and sup-ported in maintaining competence to meet the healthcare needs of people in their care.

RECRUITMENT AGENCIES

In addition to NHS Professionals there are various private recruiters. These agencies provide similar opportunities to NHS Professionals, but their fierce competitiveness may mean higher pay grades. It is important that you check the reputation, terms and conditions of employment offered. Recruitment agencies can exert subtle pressure making it difficult to refuse a shift despite not feeling fully confident. Do not feel pushed to accept last minute shifts where you may be out of your depth. Take care, too, to be fully aware of holiday entitlement and potential impact on pay, tax and pension allowances. You can register with more than one agency which will afford you more choice and flexibility. However, you will need to very organised in your communica-tions with each agency to avoid double bookings or confusion. A recruitment agency may require you to travel to various sites to cover shifts and this will have additional cost implications. You may also find that alignment to a particular area leads to you being 'poached' by the NHS. This may sound positive; however, it is important to be aware how tied you are to the recruiter? What does your contract say? Are you fixed to the agency for a certain timeframe? As always, the small print is important!

THE INDEPENDENT SECTOR

This is a very wide area, offering many possibilities outside the sphere of the NHS and across a diverse range of settings and clients. Independent health providers work in conjunction with the NHS and provide a vast range of care and services to NHS patients and self-funding patients across acute, primary, community, homecare, dentistry and diagnostic services. The demand and provision have increased year on year as has the cost with 14 billion pounds spent in 2020/21 which was two billion pounds more than the previous year (British Medical Association (BMA) 2022).

These settings are considered more aesthetically pleasing with better work environments and lower staff–client ratios than the NHS. However, this must be measured against the breadth and depth of experience available within the NHS. As with the agency work, it is essential to consider all the options and conditions. Working within the independent sector can be a contentious mixed bag in terms of annual increment or pay rises. Crucially maternity and sick leave are not uniform across this sector as it does not operate under the NHS Agenda for Change (NHS 2022). In independent settings you may find that these benefits are minimal or statutory and may need to be negotiated every step of the way. So, whilst better working conditions, or a Monday to Friday pattern of working with weekends off, are attractive, there can be hidden pitfalls in the long term.

INDEMNITY INSURANCE

It is mandatory for registered nurses to have indemnity insurance in place (NMC 2018). As an NHS or independent sector employee you will be covered vicariously via your organisation. However, it is your responsibility to ensure that you are covered appropriately for your role and scope of practice. If you choose to start with agency work, you are considered self-employed and will need to source your own indemnity either through a professional body or through one of the various commercial providers available.

PRECEPTORSHIP

In your first role following re-entry to the NMC register, you may need a period of preceptorship from an established nurse colleague. Drawing on the expertise of a preceptor is fundamental with research showing that most nurses who access this support find it helps to increase their confidence and competence (Marks-Maran et al. 2013). Most would agree that feeling supported and socialised are key factors in a successful transition into the workplace.

The NHS recognises the value of supporting newly registered staff in their initial post-registration phase. However, preceptorship comes in many guises. When you start work, you may find a planned coordinated programme in place with prearranged access and off duty scheduled accordingly. At times, pressures on staffing can challenge this provision. Roll-on roll-off training pathways can be helpful as they offer flexibility in terms of the frequency of training and the specialist skills that can be acquired for different clinical areas. In addition, most practice settings provide flexible routes for preceptorship through distance learning via e-learning modules. Role models and peer support are still evaluated very positively, although of course a positive relationship between preceptor and preceptee is paramount to the success of this liaison. The variation in who we learn from has clear benefits because it offers broader perspectives on how situations can be approached and managed, providing opportunities to observe a wide range of skills and problem-solving capabilities. Overall, an effective preceptorship programme paves the way for lifelong learning and has a positive impact on retention (Woodruff 2017; Barrett 2020).

In Chapter 6 we discussed the emotional labour of nursing and the influence of our own well-being on how we approach the care of others. Remember that organisations have responsibilities when it comes to maintaining safe and nurturing environment. As you go through the early challenges of a new job, the provision of this ongoing support should be visible. Part of self-care and compassion lies in making good choices about where you work. It is important that the organisation and team is the right fit for you just as you need to be the right fit for the role.

CULTURAL COMPETENCE AND CULTURAL HUMILITY

Nowadays most countries are multicultural with diverse populations and communities. This has had a big impact on health and social care provision, delivery and staffing. You will already be aware of the multinational mix amongst colleagues and patients, and the need to be able to interact and negotiate on many levels to ensure good therapeutic and working relationships. As a returner you are likely to have acquired experience of different scenarios in other areas of work. You may be thinking back on past situations that made you feel uncomfortable and realise now that you may have handled something differently. The terms 'cultural competence' and 'cultural humility' embrace the approaches and attributes required to maintain equality and understanding with different groups of people.

Cultural competence is defined as having the attitude, knowledge and skills to work and deliver care to and with diverse populations (Seelman et al. 2017).

Saha (2018) outline key components that a healthcare organisation can put in place to enable cultural competence. These are:

- A diverse workforce that reflects the local community.
- Local and accessible services from all points of view including language assistance.
- Continuous staff training to ensure ongoing awareness of appropriate services and to raise confidence in recognising and addressing bias and stereotyping.

Cultural competence and person-centred care are embedded within our professional code (NMC 2018). Poor experiences of care in the past can impact on how people engage with health services in the future. It is vital to respect and understand cultural contexts as this helps us to understand health behaviours and the choices people make. Within the profession the expectation that care is person centred also places greater focus on equality and diversity. DeSantis (1994) suggests that when a nurse interacts with a patient there is a meeting of three cultures – the nurse's professional culture, including values, beliefs and practices; the patient's cultural life experience of sickness and health and his or her own values and beliefs; and the culture of the setting in which the encounter takes place (be it hospital, community or family residence). Although arguably somewhat fixed or outmoded, there are useful reminders in DeSantis' viewpoint.

More recently, the term 'cultural humility' has come to the fore. This reflects a more dynamic ethos which moves away from knowing towards a position of learning. We are encouraged to perceive our own biases and develop insight into the disparities and discrimination that may exist within minority groups. 'Cultural humility refers to an orientation towards caring for one's patients that is based on: self-reflexivity and assessment, appreciation of patents' expertise on the social and cultural context of their lives, openness to establishing power-balanced relationships with patients, and a lifelong dedication to learning' (Lekas et al. 2020, p. 2).

In the following account a returning health visitor demonstrates her sensitivity and wide understanding of the potential for cultural misunderstandings during a primary visit.

Returner's Account

I telephoned a family whose ethnicity was Polish to arrange a primary visit. There was no indication on the client record that the family needed an interpreter to be present. However, the United Kingdom has an increasing culturally diverse society and nurses need to be aware of their patient's communication needs (Childs et al. 2009). Barrett et al. (2004) acknowledge principal factors affecting the communication process are power, race, inequalities and gender and that these result in practitioners often making short cuts, especially with clients whose first language is not English. Whilst arranging the visit time, it was obvious that the father spoke good English; however, I was unsure of his wife's understanding. I therefore offered them either the presence of a professionally trained interpreter, or the use of an interpreter service via the telephone. The father declined the offer and stated they did not need it but thanked me for asking.

At the visit I introduced myself, smiling at them and offering my congratulations as they celebrated being parents for the first time. Balzar-Riley (2008) suggests that using a friendly expression, good eye contact and open body language creates warmth and helps to build rapport. Positioning and space are also key factors and, as the mother was sitting at the top of the bed and the father was leaning against the bedroom wall, I asked permission to sit at the end of the bed. Childs et al. (2009) suggest that lack of cultural space between professional and patient can be misread as intrusive and standing above patients can be intimidating and may cause the patient to become defensive. During the consultation I was informed by the mother that she was mix feeding her infant. I asked openly if there were reasons why she had decided to mix feed. When used well, open questioning is usually considered polite and respectful, allowing individuals to express their feelings and motivations (Rollnick et al. 2008). At this point I became aware that I needed to be sensitive and resist the 'righting reflex', one of four core guiding principles of Motivational Interviewing (MI) (Rollnick et al. 2008), and not jump in stating 'Breast is Best'. As humans we possess an instinctive character to be resistant to persuasion, especially when advised to correct a course of action. Being self-aware and understanding one's own reaction to circumstances is fundamental to improving communications (Childs et al. 2009). The mother informed me that she 'felt reassured knowing what her infant had taken' and that 'she was not as unsettled after being fed formula milk'. The father interjected stating that his wife needed to sleep. Mum further stated that she didn't think she had enough milk to feed her infant sufficiently and had experienced problems getting her infant to attach to the breast. This culminated in her infant becoming distressed which was obviously increasing anxiety levels of parents.

I used the second and third core guiding principle of MI to understand the parents' motives for their decision making. I remained silent and actively listened with empathic interest, exploring their feelings through sensitive questioning, then reflecting back to ensure I had understood their reasoning. This style of communication was aimed at helping them to feel empowered to make the right choice for them (McCabe and Timmons 2013). Empowerment is the fourth guiding core principle. I explained to parents that it is normal for their infant to communicate by crying and displaying feeding cues and normal for her to want to feed regularly at the breast as she only has a tiny tummy at this stage of her development. I explained that formula milk takes longer to digest which would give the impression the infant was more satisfied for a longer period with this type of feed compared to breast milk (United Nations International Children's Emergency Fund (UNICEF) 2016). I then gently asked the mother if she wanted to establish her breastfeeding to which she replied that she did. Shifting the emphasis from a directional approach to a guiding approach is also key to implementing Baby Friendly standards, evidence-based national guidelines launched jointly by UNICEF and the World Health Organisation and demonstrated to be highly effective in improving breastfeeding practices (UNICEF & WHO 2006).

It became obvious to me the infant in question was displaying feeding cues and I asked mother if she would like me to assist her in positioning her baby to breastfeed. She agreed. After several minutes of encouragement and re-positioning, the infant successfully latched on, and the mother continued to breastfeed throughout the visit. Good communication cannot be stressed enough as a core clinical skill particularly in the influence it can have on the client's emotional health and symptom resolution (Leonard 2017). Mother has now managed to successfully breastfeed her infant for the last eight weeks. In conclusion, I have reflected positively on this experience of delivering health promotion and feel that, by taking a gentle patient-centred and motivational approach and observing cultural sensitivities, I was able to share evidence-based information which enabled behaviour change and alleviated stress for the mother, father and infant.

Whilst the health visitor's initial thoughts about language barriers or cultural differences seem to reflect cultural competence, her actions go beyond this to show cultural humility. Her words show that she is learning and adapting through the encounter. She perceives and silences her own urge to quickly correct the mixed feeding regime, aware that communication issues can push practitioners to make short cuts. Instead, her chief concerns are framed within the nurturing of a therapeutic relationship where listening and empathy take precedence. Although away from health visiting practice for quite some time, this returner's depth of understanding and skilled responses mark the merging together of recently refreshed knowledge and skills with many years of previous healthcare experience.

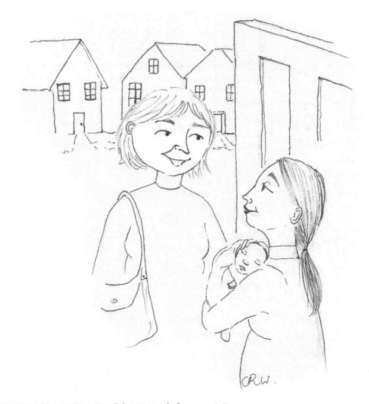

ILLUSTRATION NO. 8.1B   Health Visitor's home visit.

NMC PERSONAL RE-VALIDATION AND YOUR CONTINUING PROFESSIONAL DEVELOPMENT

Nursing involves lifelong learning with every day bringing new encounters and challenges. Continuing Professional Development (CPD) is described as the 'way in which a worker continues to learn and develop throughout their career, keeping their skills and knowledge up to date and ensuring that they can work safely and effectively' (HEE 2016). As we know, nurses have a personal and professional responsibility to identify gaps in knowledge and take steps to maintain their currency.

Once you have been admitted to the register it is essential to demonstrate that you are safe, contemporary and evidence-based in your delivery of care. This happens through the process of revalidation, introduced by the NMC in 2016. Initially, this new system was met with contention because the undercurrents of implied scrutiny were felt to undermine professional integrity. Nonetheless it has become norm and, in 2012, the General Medical Council (GMC 2012) brought in a similar process for doctors, requiring that they provide objective assurance of fitness for practice. However, revalidation for nurses is not about fitness to practice. It is a strategy to help you demonstrate that you are a safe, competent and reflective practitioner. As a registrant you are required to revalidate every three years, providing evidence of 450 practice hours or 900 hours, if dual registered. There is also a requirement to produce evidence of reflection related to events in practice and 35 hours of continuous professional development over the preceding three years. You will be notified at least 60 days prior to your revalidation due date. Here is a breakdown of what you will be asked to prepare:

- Five pieces of practice-related feedback
- Five written reflective accounts
- Written confirmation of a face-to-face reflective discussion with another NMC registrant
- Declaration of health and character
- Professional indemnity

There are various resources and templates provided by the NMC who suggest that the process of revalidation promotes a culture of 'sharing, reflection and improvement' (NMC 2016). It is recommended that we view this process as continuous one with which we should engage throughout the three-year period. We are encouraged to think of it as an opportunity to reflect on what we have achieved and set new goals.

Revalidation requires an element of organisation and planning. It is important to maintain accurate records of CPD, completing the learning formats and recording how experiences have influenced your practice. Remember learning happens every day and is not necessarily just connected to formal teaching. Chapter 5 showed how reflection helps us to unpick uncertain or challenging occurrences with a view to furthering our understanding. Try to continue what you have started during your return journey, honing your reflective skills by noting what feels significant in your everyday practice, and identifying points for future learning and potential change. The more you invest in this reflective process the more you will gain from it.

The knowledge, skills and experiences gained throughout life and career will enhance the unique tapestry that is you, as an individual and a registered nurse. We close with the thoughts of returners as they take the next steps of their journey.

Words of Wisdom on going back...

I am going back to a job I love and which I am qualified to do. This is just something for me and I loved it more than I anticipated. I feel a renewed enthusiasm for nursing. I am returning to my passion.

...and on being back

The world is your oyster when you complete the RTP course. You will have a wide choice of nursing jobs to apply for. Currently demand for nurses outstrips supply, so it is likely you will be able to negotiate days and hours to suit your home life. You will have a job for life and endless opportunities to diversify or train further.

When I completed the course, I applied for a Practice Nursing role. I negotiated part-time hours at a supportive, professionally run GP practice. There were challenges in learning so many new clinical skills, but the initial discomfort has proved well worth it. I have since completed the Practice Nursing course (fully funded) and am now enjoying being a treatment room nurse. After a twenty-year break from nursing, I am back giving care to patients as part of a great clinical team.

I love being a nurse again after all these years and enjoy the ready appreciation that you receive from patients. It feels like such a privileged role.

REFERENCES

Balzer-Riley, J. (2008). *Communication in Nursing*, 6e. Kansas: Mosby Elsevier.

Barrett, S., Komaromy, C., Robb, M. and Rogers, A. (2004). *Communication, Relationships and Care*. Routledge. The Open University.

Barrett, R. (2020). Changing preceptorship to achieve better quality training and less attrition in newly qualified nurses. *British Journal of Nursing* 29 (12): 706–709.

Benner, P. (2001). *From Novice to Expert. Excellence and Power in Clinical Nursing Practice*, Commemorative Edition. New Jersey: Prentice Hall Health.

British Medical Association (BMA) (2022). Outsourced: the role of the independent sector in the NHS.

Childs, L.L., Coles, L., and Marjoram, B., (2009). *Essential Skills Clusters for Nurses-Theory for Practice.* Chichester: Wiley-Blackwell.

DeSantis, L. (1994). Making anthropology clinically relevant to nursing care. *Leading Global Nursing Research* 20 (4): 707–715.

General Medical Council (2012). *Ready for Revalidation: Supporting Information for Appraisal and Revalidation.* London: General Medical Council. https://www.gmc-uk. org/-/media/documents/guidance---revalidation---revalidation-guidance-for-doctors_ pdf-54232703.pdf (accessed 14th June 2022).

HEE (2016). HEE (2015) Workforce plan for England: proposed education and training commissions for 2015/16.

Lekas, H.M., Pahl, K., and Fuller Lewis, C. (2020). Rethinking cultural competence: shifting to cultural humility. *Health Services Insights* 13: 1–4.

Leonard, P. (2017). Exploring ways to manage healthcare professional-patient communication issues. *[online] Support Care Cancer* 25 (Suppl.1): 7–9.

Marks-Maran, D., Ooms, A., Tapping, J. et al. (2013). A preceptorship programme for newly qualified nurses: a study of preceptees' perceptions. *Nurse Education Today* 33 (11): 1428–1434.

McCabe, C. and Timmins, F. (2013). *Communication skills for Nursing Practice,* 2e. Palgrave Macmillan.

NHS (2022). Agenda for change. https://www.healthcareers.nhs.uk/working-health/ working-nhs/nhs-pay-and-benefits/agenda-change-pay-rates/agenda-change-pay-rates

NHS Digital (2021). *NHS Vacancy Statistics England April 2015 – June 2021 Experimental Statistics – NHS Digital.* NHS Digital.

NMC (2016). Revalidation/Resources: forms and templates. http://revalidation.nmc.org. uk/download-resources/forms-and-templates.

NMC (2018). *The Code. Professional Standards of Practice and Behaviour for Nurses, Midwives and Nursing Associates.* London: NMC.

Rollnick, S., Miller, W.R., and Butler, C.B. (2008). Motivational interviewing in healthcare: helping patients change behaviour. New York. London: The Guilford Press.

Royal College of Nursing (2018). Advanced level nursing practice: introduction. RCN Standards for advanced level nursing practice, advanced nurse practitioners, RCN accreditation and RCN credentialing. PDF-006894(2).pdf.

Saha, A. (2018). *Race and the Cultural Industries.* Cambridge: Polity.

Seelman, K.L., Adams, M.A., and Poteat, T. (2017). Interventions for healthy aging among mature Black lesbians: recommendations gathered through community-based research. *Journal of Women & Aging* 29 (6): 530–542.

UNICEF (2016). A guide to infant formula for parents who are bottle feeding. The health professionals' guide. [online]. Available from: https://www.unicef.org.uk/babyfriendly/ wp-content/uploads/sites/2/2016/12/Health-professionals-guide-to-infant-formula.pdf

UNICEF & WHO (2006). Baby friendly hospital initiative: Revised updated and expanded for integrated care. [online] Available from: https://www.unicef.org.uk/babyfriendly/ baby-friendly-resources/breastfeeding-resources

Woodruff, D.W. (2017). The relationship between trained preceptors' knowledge and skills and student nurses' academic success. *ERIC*. Minneapolis (MN): Capella University.

What I Have Learnt about Myself

We close with some final insights from returning nurses as they pause to reflect on their learning before taking their next steps back into registered practice.

CONFIDENCE AND COMPETENCE

My confidence has returned, and I can do the job. Practice has been a fantastic boost. If you are determined and passionate, all is possible. Even with various challenges and doubts about my own ability, I can be assertive. I need to build further on my confidence, but I am more tenacious and focused than I realised.

I still practise well. I have discovered that I have many skills that just need time to develop. Nursing has not really changed. I am caring, capable and determined.

I have learnt that it is important to be inquisitive and questioning. People look to me to delegate and lead in stressful situations. I notice when things are wrong. I am organised, and I can bring a calming effect to the ward environment. I have learnt how much I already knew.

RESILIENCE AND WELL-BEING

I am adaptable. I can exist on less sleep than I thought and still function at a good level! I was able to manage change more than I previously believed possible. I have a

Returning to Nursing Practice: Confidence and Competence, First Edition. Ros Wray and Mary Kitson.
© 2023 John Wiley & Sons Ltd. Published 2023 by John Wiley & Sons Ltd.

good memory! Studying was a challenge, but also enjoyable – I must stop procrastinating! I have learnt that I just need to be myself, relax and not worry about fitting in. I found reflection was good for me.

I FEEL VALUED AND NEEDED

I work well in a team and feel needed and valued. I made the right decision to return. People have respected my knowledge and experience.

MY PROFESSIONAL IDENTITY

I feel I am a different nurse. I have more life experience now than before and I can use this in practice. I have noticed that I am more patient, and sometimes more emotional when caring for others. Life skills and maturity make a difference. I have recovered my identity. I like myself. I feel motivated and less frightened now about finding a job.

ACHIEVEMENT AND ENJOYMENT

I still love nursing. It's never too late to return. I actually do want to go back to work and be a Health Visitor. I have enjoyed the course and I am still capable of academic work. Writing essays can be fun: I am looking forward to further study. It has been so good being with fellow nurses again: learning and sharing. This is a massive achievement! I will never let my registration lapse again!

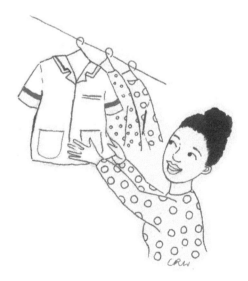

ILLUSTRATION NO. 9.1   Young mum reaching for uniform.

Index

Note: Page numbers in *italics* refer to figures.

Returning to Nursing Practice: Confidence and Competence, First Edition. Ros Wray and Mary Kitson.
© 2023 John Wiley & Sons Ltd. Published 2023 by John Wiley & Sons Ltd.